ABOUT THE AUTHORS

Dr Reg Saynor MSc, PhD, C. Chem, FRSC, FIMLS, and Member of the New York Academy of Sciences, is the Laboratory Director of the Cardiothoracic Unit, Northern General Hospital, Sheffield. He is a world authority on the 'Eskimo Diet', having directed research into the beneficial effects of fish oil on preventing heart attacks for more than twenty years. He has given interviews, lectures and held seminars on the subject throughout Europe, the United States and Canada.

Dr Frank Ryan MB, ChB(Hons), FRCP is a teaching hospital consultant physician, gastro-enterologist and consultant medical advisor to the Nutrition Institute at the Northern General Hospital, Sheffield. He has had twenty years' experience dealing with the acute management of patients with heart attacks and a long research interest in medicines. He is also the author of two novels *Sweet Summer* and *Tiger, Tiger*.

⊱THE⊰
ESKIMO DIET

How to Avoid a Heart Attack

Dr Reg Saynor
and Dr Frank Ryan

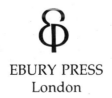

EBURY PRESS
London

For our patients who placed their trust in us and who gave kind permission to describe their very personal experiences in this book.

First published in 1990 by Ebury Press
an imprint of Century Hutchinson Ltd
20 Vauxhall Bridge Road
London SW1V 2SA

Reprinted 1990

British Library Cataloguing in Publication Data
Saynor, Reg
 The eskimo diet.
 1. Man. Heart. Coronary diseases. Prevention
 I. Title II. Ryan, Frank
 616.12305

 ISBN 0–85223–809–6

Phototypeset in Palatino by Textype Typesetters, Cambridge
Printed and bound in Great Britain by
Mackays of Chatham, Plc, Kent

Mortality from coronary heart disease has not been noticeably influenced by the expenditure of time, money and manpower on coronary ambulances, coronary care, coronary surgery, and rehabilitation. The only ways we shall make any real impact on the disease will be to prevent it or to find a way of curing it. Cure is not only likely to be unattainable but would not help to prevent the sudden deaths that account for half the fatal cases unless screening for presymptomatic coronary disease could be made more successful and could be generally applied. Prevention is the better option and it should be applied on nation-wide rather than individual scales.

Editorial, British Medical Journal

All my years of study into the mechanisms that cause coronary heart disease, together with disease of the arteries, point to diet as the major, fundamental factor.

Professor Gerald Shaper, Director of the British Regional Heart Study for the British Heart Foundation.

Contents

Acknowledgments

Foremost, we thank our wives, Margaret and Barbara, for the invaluable advice and assistance they have given us in the writing of this book. We also thank our colleagues, Mr Tim Gillott and Dr David Dawson, who shouldered the extra burden of clinical responsibility while we wrote it, and Miss Sue Willingham for her expert guidance in the dietary section.

A special thank-you to Professor Walter Bartley, who opened those vital early doors, and to Dr Hugh Sinclair for the hospitality at his Oxford home and for the contacts by letter and at meetings, when his wit and dedication have been nothing less than an inspiration.

We are grateful also to very many other colleagues for help and encouragement both in the writing of the book and over the years of clinical work and research that led to it. These include Dr David Verel, Dr David Oakley, Dr James Fleming, Mr Stuart Reed, Dr Ray Rice, Dr Willem vas Dias, Mr Clive Dixon, Dr Michael Weston, Dr Paul Rylance, Professor Gustav Born, Professor Michael Oliver, Professor Barry Lewis, Professor Robert Ackman, Professor Bruce Holub, Dr Paul Miller, Dr Paul Durrington, Dr Rudolph Riemersma, Dr Susan Barker, the late Dr Maurice Stone, Dr William S Harris, Dr Kenneth Carroll, Dr Margerita Thorngren, Dr Jorn Dyerberg, Dr Gerard Hornstra, Dr Tom Sanders, Dr David Horrobin, Dr Geoffrey Walsh, and Miss Ann Richardson.

We are indebted to the authors and publishers, who

very kindly gave us permission to refer to and quote from the following copyright sources:

Coronary Heart Disease: Risks and Reasons by Professor A G Shaper, published by Current Medical Literature in association with Duncan, Flockhart & Co Ltd.

Coronary Heart Disease Prevention: Action in the UK 1984–1987, published by The Health Education Authority.

Guide to Healthy Eating, published by The Health Education Authority.

Provisional tables on the content of omega-3 fatty acids and other fat components of selected foods, published in *The Journal of the American Dietetic Association*, June 1986, *86*, pp 788–793.

Dietary omega-3 fatty acids and mortality in the MRFIT, presented to the Second International Congress on Preventative Cardiology, 1989, by Dr Therese A Dolecek, Assistant Professor, Public Health Sciences, The Bowman Grey School of Medicine, Wake Forest University, North Carolina.

Introduction:
Why Should We Want to Write This Book?

There have been many other books and articles written about diet in relation to heart attacks, so why should we inflict yet another upon the long-suffering public? We had one reason – to give the ordinary man and woman in the street the information he or she needs to cut down to the bare minimum the risk of a heart attack.

Why write the book now? Because new information has just become available that would greatly help to reduce that risk – information that we consider to be vitally important, and which to our knowledge is simply not available from any other source at present.

No field in medicine is advancing so rapidly as our knowledge and understanding of what causes heart attacks – as the media are only too well aware. But very often useful facts are presented in such baffling scientific jargon that a potentially very interested public takes one look and then closes its eyes in incomprehension. Who could blame them for being confused, given the raw soup of half-truths and misleading stories that they pick up from colleagues and friends, into which is stirred a constant stream of bewilderment from articles in magazines and newspapers. 'Poly fats "bad for you"', 'Cold cheer for weak hearts': these were just two headlines in the course of a single week in one highly respectable newspaper. The articles below then ranged from a suggestion that all the precautions we had been taking for years on butter and saturated fats were erroneous, to extolling the merits of a kilt without 'troosers'!

Heart attacks affect all levels of society and there is a cogent need for a simple book to cover the entire subject. It's no good becoming a hypochondriac forever worrying about the demon cholesterol. No more can we pin all our hopes on the single act of giving up smoking. For goodness' sake, let's get back to good common sense! There is surely only one logical approach: to give the whole story in a clear and concise way so that you, the reader, can truly understand what it is all about. There is no need to make food a bore to prepare and unappetizing to eat. We shall show you how to reduce the risk of a heart attack considerably, while putting the joy of good eating back on to your dining table.

The major concept behind this book is that fish oil, and the importance of oily fish in our diet, is one of the most significant nutritional discoveries of the century. Our intention is to explain this discovery to you – to explain it as only experts who have been at the heart of the research from the very early days *can* explain it. We shall tell you exactly how to change your diet, what kind of fish to eat, and how to supplement what you eat with perfectly safe fish oil or capsules. And you can do all of this without making your diet boring – on the contrary, you will be making it all the more varied and exciting.

The story we have to tell is not only wonderful but scientifically accurate and true. We are responsible doctors and medical scientists – not characters jumping on the bandwagon of popular fears and phobias. At the same time, we have no intention of complicating the issue with scientific pie charts, chemical formulae and graphs – although simple drawings will be included to clarify the explanation.

The frightening statistics

We are most grateful to the National Forum for Coronary Heart Disease Prevention for permission to quote from their lucid and timely book, *Coronary Heart Disease Prevention – Action in the UK 1984–1987*, published by the Health Education Authority:

In the second half of the twentieth century, coronary heart disease has seriously affected the life expectancy and health of the UK population. It has also been responsible for many strokes and cases of peripheral arterial disease. In 1985 in the UK, 186,000 deaths were registered for coronary heart disease ... [which] is the commonest cause of death in men for every age decade from 45 upwards. In women it is the second commonest cause of death, after all cancers [i.e. all cancers of any part of the body put together] for ages 45–74 and the commonest cause of death from age 75 upwards. The situation is particularly serious in middle age. For instance, in 1985 coronary heart disease accounted for 39 per cent of all deaths in men aged 55–64 and 23 per cent of all deaths in women in the same age group.

There can be no doubting the importance of the subject.

One in three of the male population of the United Kingdom will eventually suffer from coronary artery disease. It accounts for more than a quarter of the total death rate in both men and women. One in five dies during a heart attack, and the total incidence of heart attacks has been estimated at between 500,000 and 800,000 per year; from these figures the huge importance of this illness in our lives becomes immediately apparent. These appalling statistics rage throughout the most cultured nations of the world, including the countries of western and eastern Europe, the United States, Canada, Australia, New Zealand and South Africa, and the disease is increasing rapidly even in the Third World. In the United States, more than a million people a year suffer heart attacks and more than half a million die as a result.

Oh, well – it's only old age creeping on, isn't it? No – most certainly not! A heart attack is very often fatal at a comparatively young age. One in five men below retirement age will suffer a heart attack, and one in ten will die from it; it is also now increasing rapidly as a cause of death in women. Frankly it terrifies all of us, making us desperate to discover some means of avoiding this catastrophe. Yet it isn't fate – it need not happen!

Here in the UK, particularly in Scotland and Northern Ireland, we have the unenviable star spot at the top of the list, having the highest incidence of death from heart attack per hundred thousand population in the world. Twenty years ago we shared this deadly position with Australia, Canada, the United States and New Zealand. But thanks to changes in their lifestyles, the inhabitants of these countries have considerably reduced their death rate from heart attacks. Why? Take a single sad statistic. In the UK only 5 per cent of the population ever bothers (or is encouraged) to have its blood fats checked. But in the United States, for example, more than half the population does this regularly.

Heart attacks are nothing other than an extremely common *disease* – a disease which, like tuberculosis in the past, can be prevented, and hopefully even eradicated one day. Meanwhile, heart attacks recognize no formal national boundary or age or sex barrier. We owe it to ourselves and our families to do all in our power to reduce the risk we run. And a most important clue to prevention lies in the fact that the disease shows marked differences in frequency throughout the world. Indeed there are communities who hardly know that a heart attack exists.

The advice given in *The Eskimo Diet* will considerably reduce the risk of your having a heart attack no matter where you live in the world, whether you are male or female, whether you smoke or you don't, no matter what awful diet you eat now – no matter even if you have had a heart attack already and all the risk factors are operating against you.

⤐ 1 ⤐

What Is a Heart Attack?

How the heart works

You don't need a science degree – or even an O-level in biology – to understand the mechanics of a heart attack. It really is very simple.

First, a word about the circulation of the blood. The heart is a pump which sends blood on its way through the body. Blood goes to the lungs to pick up oxygen from the air we breathe. This bright red oxygenated blood is then conveyed round the body in the arteries and returns to the heart, with the oxygen used up, via the veins as dark red, de-oxygenated blood. Then the cycle starts all over again.

Figure 1 is a drawing of the four chambers that make up the human heart, showing the direction of the blood flow.

The walls of these chambers are composed of a special kind of muscle which does not tire. Each side of the heart, left and right, has a thin-walled chamber called an atrium, which lies over a much bigger and stronger chamber called a ventricle. Each atrium is separated from its corresponding ventricle, which ensures that the blood flows in one direction only. The right atrium is separated from the right ventricle by the tricuspid valve; while the left atrium is separated from the left ventricle by what is called the mitral valve, because it looks like a bishop's mitre. Notice also that

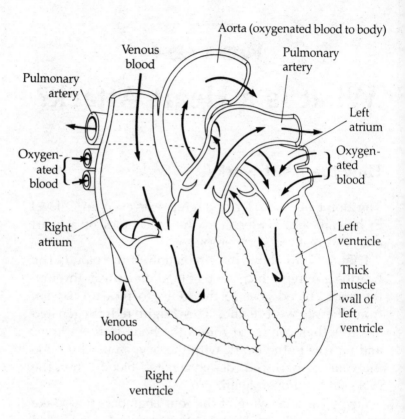

Figure 1 *The chambers of the heart*

the left ventricle has a much thicker and more powerful muscle wall than the right ventricle.

The *lub-dub* of the normal heartbeat tells you that this cycle has two components. The *lub* occurs at the end of the contraction of the two atria, which pump blood under low pressure through the mitral and tricuspid valves into the ventricles. When the ventricles are full of blood and their powerful walls start to contract, the mitral and tricuspid valves are forced shut, creating the first of the two heart sounds.

From the right ventricle de-oxygenated blood, which has been gathered in the right atrium from all the veins of the body, is now pumped into the pulmonary artery to be oxygenated in the lungs. From the left ventricle the oxygenated blood returning to the left atrium after its passage through the lungs is pumped under great pressure into the aorta, the huge artery that carries oxygenated blood to all the living tissues in the body. Each of these two major arteries also has a valve at its beginning, called respectively the pulmonary and aortic valves, so that the blood cannot go backwards as the ventricles relax. The abrupt closure of the aortic and pulmonary valves at the end of the contraction of the ventricles makes the *dub*, or second part of the heartbeat sound.

Of course there has to be a control mechanism that tells the chambers to contract – this is an electrical conducting system with living bundles that behave in an identical manner to tiny electric cables and which run over the walls of the chambers. The reason your heart beats roughly seventy-two times per minute is that there is a tiny pacemaker (called the sino-atrial node) right on top of the heart, which discharges electrically at this frequency. The signal to contract is transmitted throughout the electric-conducting tissue, so that the signal goes to exactly the right muscle cells at the right time and in a perfectly co-ordinated movement through-out the four chambers of the heart.

As you might imagine, if this electrical control of the heartbeat becomes upset the consequences can be very serious. This kind of upset is in fact responsible for many of the deaths from heart attack. This will be further explained in Chapter 3, which includes practical advice on how to reduce this risk. But for the moment, let's just concentrate on the movements of the blood.

Contrary to what you might have supposed, the heart

muscle does not get its oxygenated blood from inside the big chambers. Right at the beginning of the aorta and just above the aortic valve, the first arteries that arise from it, like tree branches, are the ones which supply the heart muscle with its oxygenated blood supply. There are two of these, left and right, which run down over the surface of the heart – you may well have seen these arteries, thick and pink, accompanied by a thin-walled blue vein, running in the fat on the surface of an ox's or pig's heart in the butcher's shop.

Figure 2   *The coronary arteries*

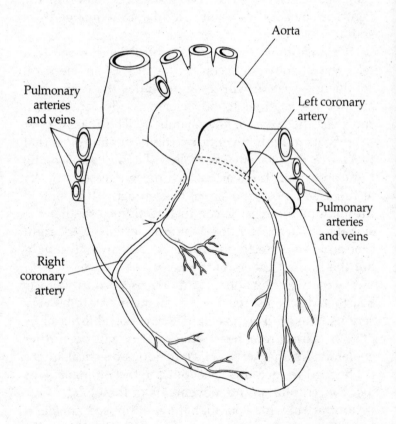

In Latin, *corona* means a crown. The coronary arteries crown the heart in more senses than one. Each of them subdivides into two main branches, so that from the point of view of a heart surgeon there are effectively four coronary arteries of great importance (see *Figure 2*). There is then a series of further subdivisions, ramifying down into the muscle wall of the heart.

How arteries get blocked

A heart attack occurs when a clot of blood blocks a coronary artery or one of its main branches. How and why does this come about?

Figure 3   *A normal artery in cross-section*

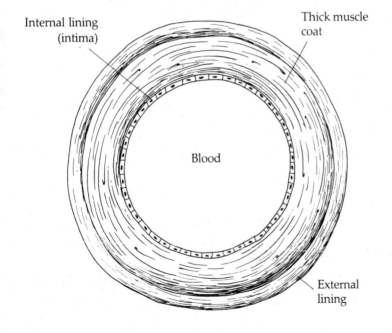

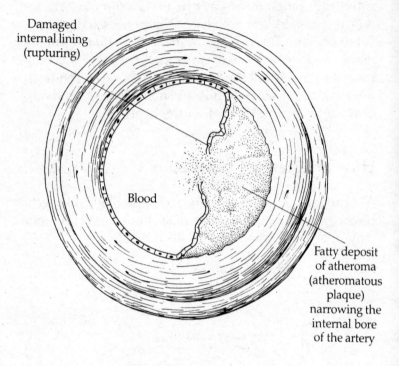

Damaged
internal lining
(rupturing)

Blood

Fatty deposit
of atheroma
(atheromatous
plaque)
narrowing the
internal bore
of the artery

Figure 4   *Artery showing deposit of atheroma*

Atheroma

The term 'atheroma' may be a mouthful, but it's even easier to understand than a heart attack. *Figure 3* shows the structure of an artery when cut in cross-section.

Notice that its wall is mainly made up of a thick muscle layer and that there is a smooth lining, called the intima, which is a membrane composed of living cells. Atheroma is the medical term used to describe the laying down of a fatty, porridge-like substance under the lining of the artery. The effect is all too clear from the drawing above (see *Figure 4*):

Why do we get these deposits of atheroma in the first

place? There will be more about this later, but basically atheroma is made up of fat, mainly cholesterol (see Chapter 4), and its deposition is partially a result of high levels of fat in our blood. It is now believed that smoking damages the living cells of the intima, and one of the bad effects of this habit is a worsening of this process of atheroma, or hardening of the arteries. The results are obvious: much less blood can pass through the artery.

The deposit is usually very uneven, with a tendency to affect arteries in very localized places; these patches of narrowing are referred to as atheromatous plaques. In the heart they give rise to the medical condition called angina.

The reason is easy to understand. If you walk uphill, or against a wind, your heart has to pump more blood to the huge muscles in your legs, and in order to achieve this the heart muscle has to work harder. All this extra work has to be done by the thick-walled and powerful left ventricle – but it means that the living muscle of the left ventricle itself will need a much richer blood supply. This is usually accommodated by increasing the number of heartbeats and by opening up (dilating) the diameter of the coronary arteries so that more blood can get through to the heart muscle. But of course if the coronary arteries have been narrowed as a result of atheroma the increased flow of blood simply cannot get through.

This lack of blood flowing to the needy heart muscle causes pain, which is a symptom of angina. The pain is identical to that of a heart attack but much less severe, and usually passes off within a few minutes of resting.

Angina and other pains

Many people worry unduly about any chest pain, assuming that it must be angina. But this is a fallacy.

Angina usually comes on *during* heavy exertion, especially walking. Walking uphill, after a heavy meal or on a cold day is particularly likely to bring on the pain. Feeling exhausted, getting out of breath, or getting a sharp pain like a stitch after reaching home is *not* the pattern of angina.

The pain is not usually sharp (although, human nature being as diverse as it is, everybody tends to get slightly different versions). It is rather a dull, heavy sensation, usually described as a tightness across the centre of the chest. In attempting to describe it, patients tend to make a fist. This pain quite frequently radiates – in other words it spreads to other parts of the body. Usually it goes into the left arm, sometimes the right arm and sometimes both; here it may feel like a numbness, a heaviness, or a tingling in the fingers. It may also rise up into the throat, where it produces a tight sensation like choking. Indeed, the term 'angina' means a choking sensation, which was how the Victorian doctors thought of it.

But for goodness' sake don't think you have heart disease because you feel a lump in your throat or have difficulty in swallowing! Perfectly healthy people get this sensation, which is termed *globus hystericus*, when they feel particularly anxious. And we all get minor aches and pains in our chest quite frequently – but they do not really fit the pattern described above and are usually nothing to worry about.

In practice, the commonest condition to be confused with heart pain, both that of angina and that of a heart attack, is indigestion arising from inflammation of the oesophagus or gullet. It is extremely common, even in young, fit people, and is characterized by a sharp pain, sometimes burning, behind the lower end of the breast bone. It is often related to stress or tension, and gets worse after a heavy meal, on bending down or when lying flat in bed at night. Unlike angina, it usually lasts for half an hour or for hours on end and may not come on while walking.

If you are at all worried that you might be getting angina, go and discuss it with your family doctor. He or she will be very familiar with this condition, which is seen in the surgery many times a day.

If your doctor diagnoses angina, don't get alarmed. It is eminently treatable, and some very effective remedies are available these days. This book will give you a great deal of useful information on the subject; but it *must* be used in conjunction with advice and therapy from your family doctor and possibly from a hospital specialist too.

Many patients may suffer from angina for years without experiencing any worsening of their condition. But there can be little doubt that angina carries with it the risk of the much more serious complication of heart attack. Most people over the age of thirty will already have some atheromatous narrowing of their coronary arteries. The first aim in our efforts to combat this disease must be to halt this process. It is never too late to reduce further narrowing and there is some evidence – as yet preliminary – that control of cholesterol and blood fats may even reverse pre-existing atheroma. The advice given in this book will certainly help you to reduce the severity of this condition. But what is of greatest concern is what happens when that artery, already somewhat narrowed by the atheromatous plaque, is suddenly filled with a blood clot, which in turn produces a heart attack (see *Figure 5*).

The risk factors

Medical research has uncovered a number of major risk factors. The important ones, already mentioned, are smoking and excess fat in the bloodstream. Smoking not

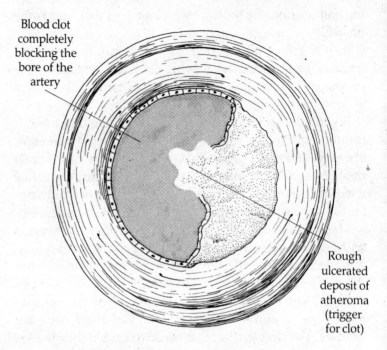

Blood clot completely blocking the bore of the artery

Rough ulcerated deposit of atheroma (trigger for clot)

Figure 5   *The clot of blood blocking an artery*

only worsens atheroma, but also promotes the blood clot which blocks the artery. Certain families have a hereditary tendency to very high fat levels in their blood; as a result they suffer much more atheroma and at a very early age. Over the last twelve years Dr Ryan has tested the blood fats of patients under the age of fifty-five who were admitted to his acute medical wards with heart attacks: the majority had raised fat levels in their blood. This is eminently treatable.

A study reported in the *British Medical Journal* some ten years ago pointed to a vague illness preceding the heart attack by up to a year, and many of the symptoms reported by case studies suggested stress. There is a medical condition called Gaisbock's syndrome, in which stress in middle-aged men makes the blood thicker, promotes a higher viscosity to its passage through the arteries (higher viscosity means an increased sluggishness to flow and hence a greater tendency to clot), and is associated with an increased incidence of heart attacks. There may be changes in the blood clottability, which links to a protein called fibrinogen, itself a vital component of the clot that blocks the artery. Cigarette smoking tends also to be associated with a more dangerous level of fibrinogen. Raised blood pressure too is connected with a higher risk. It is now believed that an increase in the stickiness of the platelets in our blood may be a vital trigger for the fatal clot – the platelets are little sticky bodies that circulate along with the red and white blood cells, and stick together like blobs of glue as a vital first component of a clot forming within the coronary arteries.

Men are more prone to heart attacks than women; indeed, before the menopause women rarely get the disease. However, in the last fifteen years postmenopausal women have seen a massive increase in their risk of getting a heart attack – so much so that women now account for 40 per cent of the total death rate from this cause. This staggering figure is probably related both to increased smoking and to the stresses resulting from the more liberated roles that women now enjoy (which often means going out to work as well as doing the housework – two jobs rather than one).

The effect of the clot in the artery

But let's return to the heart attack itself – what is the effect on the heart of the coronary artery being blocked by a blood clot? The muscle wall of the left ventricle is suddenly deprived of its blood supply. It immediately registers a pain, very similar to that of angina, but much more severe. Part of the muscle may actually die – but this takes hours to happen, vital hours during which modern medicine may be able to stop and even reverse the process. Certainly the damaged heart cannot perform its function properly; it tends to fail, and the sufferer feels suddenly very sick and breathless. The left ventricle hasn't got the strength to pump blood round the body properly and so the patient feels exhausted, unable to do anything, and usually lies down. Adrenalin pours into the blood, causing the skin to go very pale and to sweat heavily.

Thinking ahead

The basic pathological process is all too easily understood – and it *is* frightening. It frightens doctors, too, because they run just as much of a risk of heart attack as their patients do. The main purpose of this book, however, is not to frighten, but to help people avoid the situation happening in the first place. Yet even when a man or woman is in the middle of a heart attack, something new and wonderful has become possible as a result of advances in medical understanding and treatment.

Chapter 3 contains detailed practical advice on how to cope with a heart attack if you are unlucky enough to suffer one. Understanding has a most important role to play – it might well result in a smaller heart attack and therefore less likelihood of its affecting your normal lifestyle afterwards. It might even save your life.

But could there also be a single, simple treatment, nothing more than a change in our diet, that could reduce or remove all the above risk factors? It seems too good to be true, and yet there is. That treatment is the Eskimo Diet.

2

A Tale of Eskimos

In 1944 Dr Hugh Sinclair of Oxford University travelled to Canada to investigate a problem on behalf of the Canadian Air Force. By chance, during his visit the opportunity to examine Canadian Indians and Eskimos presented itself to him – as a nutritional biochemist, he had been fascinated by Eskimos and their diet for many years. His curiosity was excited by the fact that they consumed the sort of carnivorous diet that would give a cardiologist nightmares, yet they did not seem to suffer from heart attacks. That diet had the highest animal fat content of any diet in the world, because of the very high proportion of seal meat and blubber that it contained; nevertheless Eskimos were said to have low blood cholesterol levels.

It must have been tempting for Dr Sinclair to speculate, as others of his medical colleagues had done, that the Eskimos' freedom from heart attacks must have resulted from Darwinian evolution. The explanation would be along these lines. Take an isolated population such as the Eskimos. Put them all on a diet that would put them at great risk of dying from heart attacks. Over thousands of years those liable to get heart attacks would die from them and be less likely to produce children, while the more resistant would probably survive and have children. In this way, over those thousands of years, there would be a natural tendency for a population to evolve that was resistant to heart attacks in spite of their high fat consumption. This was a very reasonable explanation, and one which might easily have been correct.

Fortunately, Hugh Sinclair was not satisfied. In the best spirit of scientific enquiry, he rejected the obvious and asked himself a very different question. What if the Eskimos are essentially no different from ourselves in the Western world? What if they are just as liable to suffer heart attacks? Then there must be some other factor, something quite vital, in their environment which protects them from the great danger of their high-fat diets. The most obvious way in which their daily lives differed from those of people in the UK was that they ate a lot of fish. Could this be the explanation?

First of all Dr Sinclair checked whether the Eskimos really did have a low cholesterol level. By looking into their eyes it is possible to detect people with a tendency to high blood cholesterol. At a relatively young age they may have a white ring about the edge of the iris that is normally only found in the elderly; then it is called the *arcus senilis*, but when found in somebody under the age of sixty it is known as a premature *arcus senilis*. Hugh Sinclair looked for evidence of this amongst the Eskimos, but did not find it. No more did he find any cataracts, which are sometimes (though not always) linked to the degenerative changes caused by age in Western populations. In time other medical workers would amply confirm his findings that Eskimos are virtually free of many of the common diseases found in the Western world. The differences are fascinating.

It is not just heart attacks which Eskimos, on their traditional diet, avoid. They are also virtually free of psoriasis, bronchial asthma, diabetes, immune disorders such as an over-active thyroid, and they have a reduced risk of rheumatoid arthritis, dental decay, gallstones, appendicitis, and bowel ailments such as diverticulitis and ulcerative colitis. On the other hand they are just as prone to cancer, peptic ulcers, epilepsy, cerebral haemorrhage and mental illness.

Following his first trip to the Eskimos, Dr Sinclair moved away to continue with other scientific research; the opportunity of further study was very nearly lost in the interim, since the Eskimos' traditional way of life was gradually eroded by Westernization until it was almost extinct. However, in 1976 he was invited by two Danish scientists, Dr Hans Bang and Dr Jorn Dyerberg, to join them in an expedition to the one surviving colony in north-west Greenland where the population still consumed a diet consisting predominantly of seal meat and fish.

Since Dr Sinclair's first pioneering visit, the scientific world had become increasingly intrigued with the story of the Eskimos. What particularly interested the Danish scientists was the fact that these Eskimos, in spite of living in a harsh and hostile environment and eating their very high-fat diet, lived into a good old age, barring accidents. The research team very quickly established the first important scientific evidence against a genetic explanation for this. Eskimos who had emigrated from Greenland into eastern Canada and adopted a Western lifestyle were now suffering from heart attacks and the other diseases associated with Western living – within a single generation they had acquired just the same risk as we have.

The team was desperately keen to study the Eskimos in their natural environment before it was too late. But there is a limit to how much investigation you can perform from a makeshift laboratory perched on a dog sled. They were, however, able to collect samples of Eskimos' food, take samples of blood for later analysis, and perform some simple tests on the spot. Immediately they discovered very important differences between the Eskimos and ourselves.

If you stick a needle into your finger or the fleshy part of an ear-lobe you expect to bleed a little. The bleeding quickly stops, the time taken being called the 'bleeding time'. It is essential that blood contains factors that clot under certain circumstances or we would bleed to death from even a minor wound such as a shaving cut or the menstrual loss in a woman. The average bleeding time for the British is about four or five minutes, but in the Eskimos it was about eight minutes. Put simply, Eskimo blood does not clot as easily as ours does.

Next the scientists measured blood fats. They were puzzled by their findings, that the level of cholesterol in Eskimo blood was not in fact lower than that of Western blood. But at this time the importance of different types of cholesterol in the blood was not understood. As will be explained in Chapter 4, this is vital. The Eskimos have the same total blood cholesterol as ourselves but it is distributed in quite a different way – a much safer and more protective way than our own.

There is another very important fat in the blood – whole fat or triglyceride. On the Eskimos' diet you would expect this to be very high indeed – a big risk factor in heart attacks. On the contrary: the three researchers found that the blood triglyceride was much lower in Eskimos than in ourselves. This seemed inexplicable. The researchers probed further.

Our blood contains tiny particles called platelets, rather like sticky little specks of biological gum. Their role is to gather at a site of bleeding, stick to the damaged blood vessel walls and plug the hole. This is the first and most vital process in our bodies for the formation of blood clots. In the Eskimos' blood it was found that these platelets had less of a tendency than ours to form a clot.

Hugh Sinclair knew that all these differences were of great importance. Yet he had to convince the world that they were related to the Eskimos' diet and were not a result of genetic differences between the Eskimos and ourselves. So he decided to conduct a somewhat hazardous experiment. Back in Oxford, he decided he would put himself and some other volunteers on to the Eskimos' diet. But as so often happens in the most innovative of scientific experiments, when he realized that seal meat might contain hazardous substances he felt he had to go it alone.

It wasn't until March 1979 that he managed to obtain a deep-frozen seal. For a hundred days he lived on a diet of boiled seal meat, fish, crustaceans, molluscs and water. He carefully weighed and recorded all the foods he used, weighed himself daily and waited for things to happen.

His weight fell from 15 stone to 13 stone 2 lb – although this is not a manner of slimming that we would recommend! His bleeding time increased from a normal four minutes to fifty minutes, but then restabilized at fifteen minutes. This change was so dramatic that it resulted in nose-bleeds and bruising; obviously he was overdoing things. Whatever factor was present in the Eskimo diet that had an effect on the clotting of the blood, he was administering to himself in excess. Readers should be reassured that on the Eskimo Diet recommended in the later chapters of this book there is no danger whatsoever of this happening.

Over this period Hugh Sinclair measured his blood fats, and experienced a decrease in his blood triglycerides exactly as found in the Eskimos. His blood cholesterol increased slightly, but he discovered that this was accompanied by a significant rise in the 'protective cholesterol' (known as HDL–cholesterol, which will be explained in Chapter 4). His platelets also showed the same reduced tendency to clot as he had earlier found in the Eskimos. In other words he had proved that all the differences in heart attack risk factors, the benefits the Eskimos enjoyed compared to ourselves, were a result of their diet. It was a momentous discovery.

Until that point, doctors had taken a rather simplistic attitude to diet, particularly to the diet eaten in the developed nations. A great deal of work had been undertaken earlier, particularly with regard to vitamins, but the overall attitude – and it still prevails today – was that the main problem was over-eating. It is indeed true that we eat too much of many foods in our diet and this makes us liable to such conditions as diabetes. Over-eating is also an important factor in heart disease, particularly with regard to our high intake of saturated fats. This book does not under-estimate this well-proven association and sound advice on this aspect of diet will be given in later chapters.

It is, however, unfortunate that over-concentration on the 'too much' hypothesis, particularly with regard to cholesterol, has blinded us to the possibility that there might be another vitally important risk factor in connection with heart attacks. The very confusion that rages about the real risk of cholesterol, polyunsaturates versus monounsaturates, and so on, should have alerted the scientific world to the fact that some vital part of the explanation was missing. The differences of opinion amongst eminent researchers have done nothing but cloud the picture, while, even after huge changes in diet that have often destroyed our real enjoyment of food, it is still not certain whether all of this has significantly reduced the risk of heart attacks. It has not occurred to us in our affluent society that there was an additional 'too little' risk factor in our diet.

Now the research of Hugh Sinclair and his colleagues was suggesting something radically different. While we might well be eating too much meat and animal fat (although considerably less than the Eskimos!), it was probably of even greater significance that we were not eating enough fish. There was already a great deal of circumstantial evidence to corroborate this. In the nineteenth and early twentieth centuries, when fish formed a much larger proportion of the British diet, heart attacks were much rarer. During the Second World War, when fish consumption again rose in Britain, the incidence of heart attacks fell significantly.

Clearly the relationship between fish in the diet and the risk of heart attacks warranted a great deal more scientific investigation. From the brilliant and courageous early researches of Hugh Sinclair, the scientific baton now moved to a few key medical scientists throughout the world. It was at about this stage, in the late 1970s, that Dr Reg Saynor, in his capacity as Director of the Cardiothoracic Laboratory at the Northern General Hospital in Sheffield, became involved with the developing story of the Eskimo Diet. His work would become of global importance.

Throughout much of the book we shall be telling you how best to use the Eskimo Diet to avoid heart attacks, but since more than one in fifty adults a year has a heart attack, we must first accept that some people will continue to have heart attacks. We shall therefore give you some practical advice to reduce the risk even during a heart attack.

3

How to Cope with a Heart Attack

Nobody wants a heart attack. And prevention is really up to you. Your family doctor is in the front line – if there is something you don't understand, then don't be afraid to ask him or her about it.

If you are actually having a heart attack, however, then the place for you is a hospital and as quickly as possible. This is the true story of one of our patients, George, who is forty-five years old and works as a central heating engineer.

I got a severe pain across my chest. I would describe it as a tightness more than anything else. I thought it was similar to indigestion but it worried my wife and she called out the family doctor. I think the reason she got worried was that this kind of pain is unusual for me and she thought I looked pretty sick. The doctor came, a lady doctor, and had a look at me. She listened to my heart and my chest and didn't find anything really wrong but like my wife she didn't like the sound of the pain. She was also worried because I looked sick. It worried her enough to call an ambulance straightaway and she even sat in her car outside my house and waited for the ambulance to arrive.... I discovered later on that my heart stopped in the ambulance while they were taking me to hospital. I think the total time between my first feeling the pain and getting into the ambulance was no more than thirty minutes, thanks to my wife and family doctor. Later, after Dr Ryan had explained what happened, I found out which ambulancemen had saved my life and I paid them a visit and thanked them.

This story tells us so much that is important about the emergency management of a heart attack. If George had waited only another half-hour his heart would have stopped at home – and you hardly need to be a doctor to understand what that would have meant. In his case there can be no doubt that early diagnosis and transfer to hospital were essential.

Early diagnosis means self-diagnosis

That first hour or two can be absolutely vital. Most of the people who die from heart attacks do so at home, without ever reaching hospital.

Remember what we referred to in Chapter 2, that very important electrical system which regulates the heartbeat? The pacemaker automatically fires at about seventy-two times a minute, and the signal is carried from here to every muscle cell in the wall of the heart and tells it exactly when to contract.

Imagine what happens when a part of that vital left ventricle is cut off from its blood supply as a result of a clotted coronary artery. Many muscle cells lose their oxygen supply and cannot contract properly. Of even greater importance, these damaged fibres have a tendency to fire off electrical signals themselves – in other words false pacemakers set themselves into action in wrong parts of the heart and are all firing here and there without the slightest co-ordination.

The effect on the heartbeat is disastrous. Instead of the heart contracting in a single, powerful, co-ordinated movement, little bits are wobbling at all the wrong times, so the overall effect is useless for propelling blood. A heart in this desperate state looks like a quivering bag of worms; doctors call it ventricular fibrillation. In effect the heartbeat has stopped, and within three minutes the brain will be irreversibly dead. For the majority of people who die from heart attacks, this is precisely what happens. It was this complication that was reversed by the ambulancemen in George's case.

The first very good reason for going straight into hospital if you are having a heart attack is the fact that this problem can usually be dealt with either in hospital, or, given high-tech facilities, in the ambulance en route. In 1987, the Royal College of Physicians expressed very strong concern about this complication:

The majority of cardiac arrests in the community are related to ischaemic heart disease [mainly heart attack].... Of [those] deaths 40 per cent occur within one hour of the onset of symptoms, and amongst middle-aged and younger male patients 63 per cent of the deaths occur within one hour. The majority, therefore, occur outside of hospital and over 90 per cent of these deaths are due to ventricular fibrillation which is potentially reversible.

How do I know I'm having a heart attack?

The answer may seem obvious, but the statistics suggest otherwise. It's no good knowing that hospital is the right place for someone suffering a heart attack if you can't recognize when you – or someone else – are having one. We gave a questionnaire to twenty patients immediately after their admission to hospital with a confirmed heart attack. We asked them if they realized it was a heart attack – or otherwise what made them call their doctor or dial 999. We also asked them how long it took between the start of their pain and arriving at the hospital. These are some of their answers:

Realized it was a heart attack – 11

Thought it might be but didn't want to believe it – 2

Didn't think it was a heart attack – 7

Only two patients reached hospital within half an hour of the onset of their pain. Most of the others took between two and six hours, while two out of our twenty waited a staggering forty-eight hours. This delay must be avoided if that very high death rate from ventricular fibrillation in the first hour or two after the heart attack is to be reduced.

Because of this we paid particular attention to what caused the delay. Clearly there was less danger of delay if the patient recognized that he or she was suffering a heart attack, but even then many who knew what was happening waited far too long before calling for help. When we asked those who had correctly diagnosed their own heart attacks what drew them to this conclusion, nearly all mentioned the severity and character of the pain. Many also remarked on the fact that it went down their arm or that they also felt generally sick. Two out of the eleven who recognized their pain had already had one previous heart attack.

Those patients who did not recognize their pain as likely to be caused by a heart attack most commonly attributed it to indigestion or stomach ache (although in fact their descriptions were identical in most cases to the pain described by the eleven who correctly diagnosed themselves).

Why not make this book really work for you? Mark these few pages and keep them available for easy reference.

This is what a heart attack feels like.

Chest pain

This is very similar to the pain of angina, described in Chapter 2, but it is more severe and does not go away with resting. People often say it is the worst pain they have ever experienced, including women with experience of childbirth. But there are exceptions, and elderly patients in particular may not feel as much pain. Because of its severity it should not usually be confused with indigestion or the usual sort of aches and pains we all experience in the various muscles and bones of our chest wall.

People describe it as 'a tight gripping sensation', 'a crushing sensation', 'a sensation of great heaviness or a great weight across the chest', or 'a tight band around the chest'. Note, however, that a minority have atypical pain, which they think is burning in character and similar to indigestion. This makes the heart attack much more difficult to diagnose, but an important clue is given by the severity of the pain and the other associated features described here.

The pain is usually felt, not about the left nipple or on the left-hand side of the chest, but across the centre of the chest or across the upper abdomen. It frequently moves into the arms or into the throat, and not uncommonly may move or even arise in the back. Note, however, that with these less usual sites the character of the pain (i.e. heavy, dull, constricting) tends to remain the same. In the arms it often feels like a tight band or heaviness, and tingling or numb sensations are often felt in the fingers.

Some anxious people who are just worrying about their hearts can get tingling in their fingers and feet. This is caused by breathing too deeply, without their being aware they are doing it, which has the effect of temporarily lowering the calcium in the blood.

Other features of a heart attack

The most important of these is that somebody who does not usually feel at all ill suddenly feels very sick indeed. (Anxious people tend to feel ill most of the time, and this is not at all typical of a heart attack.) The typical heart attack victim has usually felt normal until the attack begins. Then he or she will look pale, and often sweats and has cold skin. A close relative will recognize that the patient really does look and seem seriously ill. The reason for the cold, clammy look is the effects of adrenalin. This closes down the circulation to the skin and causes the patient to sweat profusely. He or she will also tend to be breathless and will feel exhausted and therefore want to lie down (although one patient climbed Snowdon on the day he had a heart attack and only called on his doctor when he arrived home the next day!).

False alarms

It will not have escaped your notice that we have taken considerable trouble to try to deflect people suffering from anxiety from imagining they are having a heart attack. The imagination can easily create a sense of choking or tightness in the throat, of not being able to take a proper breath, and of tingling in the hands and feet and about the mouth. We want to avoid the risk of family doctors and the emergency services being over-burdened by false alarms. You simply do not suffer from heart attacks every day. With a mortality of one in five in each attack, the laws of chance would be strictly against very many heart attacks in a lifetime.

Remember that the pain is usually severe and is rarely the kind a sufferer will have experienced before; it is also generally accompanied by other signs of serious illness. Don't for goodness' sake become neurotic and keep calling out your doctor with every little pain. On the other hand, if you are seriously worried, seek help immediately. If, as sometimes happens, a patient calls his or her doctor out and it isn't a heart attack, discuss it properly with the doctor and find out how your experience is different from that of a heart attack. Remember that doctors are caring and highly trained human beings but you cannot expect them to be infallible. A little communication will often save a great deal of long-term difficulty.

The British Heart Foundation publishes free booklets which will give interested readers further information on many aspects of heart disease, including the symptoms of a heart attack. The address to write to is given on page 183.

First aid

What do you do if somebody collapses when you are nearby and you cannot feel a pulse and he or she is not breathing? Time is of the essence and here's some very simple advice that might save that person's life. First of all, check there are no false teeth in their mouth and that they are not choking on their tongue. You have all of a few seconds in which to do this. Although it sounds unpleasant, it is quite easy to put your hand into their mouth until your fingers curl round the angle at the back of the tongue; then you just pull it forwards. If the airway was blocked, they will immediately start to make some breathing efforts.

If they still haven't taken a breath and you can't feel any pulse (you have just further seconds to establish this), then thump the centre of the chest over the breastbone very hard and a little faster than once a second. If you are a small person, use both fists in a ball. If you are fairly strong or heavy, use one fist. The sharp thumps may damp down the irregular heart contractions and allow the normal pacemaker to take over.

If you feel strongly motivated, find out from your directory or from your local Health Authority the telephone number of your Health Education Unit. Every health district in the UK has one. This unit will be able to put you in touch with an expert, usually a member of the St John's Ambulance, who can provide instructions on how to resuscitate somebody from a cardiac arrest. All it will take is a single two-hour session. There is gathering evidence that this kind of skill in a community really does save lives.

The coronary care unit

Although hospital is the best place to be if you have had a heart attack, it is unfortunately the case that many patients are frightened of the sort of high-technology invasion of privacy that they will experience. All sorts of mistaken beliefs and fears abound, so some reassurance is called for.

As a junior hospital doctor, Frank Ryan once worked with a colleague who was a wonderful doctor in every way except for the fact that he refused ever to visit the coronary care unit. These units are staffed by the kindest and most dedicated staff you could ever wish to meet, but this man was frightened that he would one day have a heart attack and end up as one of their patients.

Let's debunk this fear with a hefty dose of common sense. What is a coronary care unit, and why did they ever come about?

The answer lies in those terrifying statistics. During the single year 1987, 179,178 men and women died from coronary artery disease in the UK; and more than half a million men and women suffered from coronary artery disease but were not killed by it. Coronary care units arose in order to contain this terrible epidemic.

First and foremost, they are geared to prevent or treat that sudden-death complication already discussed in detail, ventricular fibrillation. They are also expert in the caring aspects of nursing. They keep the sick patient free of pain and allow him or her to get the rest that is essential in those first few alarming days after admission to hospital. There are many other very important aspects of coronary care units which we cannot go into in this book, except for one innovative treatment which is now available to every patient suffering from a heart attack.

The new clot-dissolving treatment

In 1988 the Northern General Hospital, like others throughout the United Kingdom, was taking part in a trial of a new treatment for heart attacks. Abruptly, the trial was interrupted and then cancelled. The reason was the confirmation of the important role of a new medical advance, thrombolytic therapy. It was based on a wonderful drug called streptokinase, derived from a bacterium which was once a dreaded killer of mothers in childbirth. From this fearsome bacterium was derived a chemical poison which was turned back upon itself and put to medical use. Streptokinase was the first in a line of medical treatments which, when injected intravenously, actually dissolve the clot that is blocking the coronary artery.

The medical trial which was interrupted so suddenly was the evaluation of this new line of treatment – testing if it was of benefit to patients who had just arrived in hospital with a heart attack. Those patients receiving the new thrombolytic or clot-dissolving treatment were benefiting much more than those who did not, and it was therefore considered unethical to continue with the comparison. It was decided that all patients should be considered for this new wonder therapy.

But here again time was important. This therapy works best when a heart attack is very recent indeed – another very powerful reason for early self-diagnosis and admission to hospital.

Roy, a sixty-two-year-old caretaker, was given this treatment in a coronary unit. His words may help to reassure those people who feel a little apprehensive about entering this high-technology scene.

On 24 June I had one or two dizzy attacks and then I started to get an aching pain in my shoulder and arms. This gradually got worse over three days. At first it got better when I rested, but then resting did not get rid of the pain. I went in to work but after finishing the morning shift the pain got worse and came on in more frequent attacks, and I thought it was my old stomach trouble and I was making too much acid. I then had a very bad attack with pains in the chest and down my arms and I asked my wife to telephone for an ambulance, which came within minutes and I was admitted to hospital. I was wired up to an electrocardiogram and told I had had a heart attack and was put on coronary care.... Once they had given me an injection I felt a lot better. I thought the coronary care unit was marvellous. You couldn't get better treatment if you were royalty. All the time the nurses were asking me if I was all right. They never ignored me for one minute.

The role of surgery

This book would not be complete without some words on surgery and heart attack rehabilitation. In recent years there has been a mushrooming of high-technology procedures for dealing with coronary atherosclerosis. The once rare operation, coronary artery bypass grafting (cabbage or CABG grafting) is now a standard treatment for patients with either severe angina or a number of other indications. The changes we have seen in the Northern General Hospital are typical of what is happening countrywide and internationally. By the end of 1989, a team of four cardiac and cardiothoracic surgeons which included Professor Geoffrey Smith had performed a staggering 350 of these operations in that year alone. So what exactly does this famous operation consist of?

The surgeon removes a length of vein from the leg and then uses this vein in a grafting operation which bypasses the areas of severe narrowing in the coronary arteries. Usually anything from two to four arteries (or even more) need grafting at once. The drawing (see *Figure 6*) shows how this is done. By grafting the vein between the start of the aorta and bypassing the narrowed portion of the coronary artery a good supply of blood is allowed to flow through to the muscle of the heart once more.

What is an exercise electrocardiogram?

Otherwise known as a 'stress test' or a 'treadmill test', this is an electrocardiogram which is performed during exercise. Very often if you are suffering from angina, the electrocardiogram (ecg) will be normal when you are lying down and so little will be learnt from a resting or normal ecg. During graded exercise, the normal resting ecg will often become abnormal ('ischaemic'), and the amount of exercise needed to cause it to become ischaemic provides very useful information on the severity of the disease in the coronary arteries. This test is

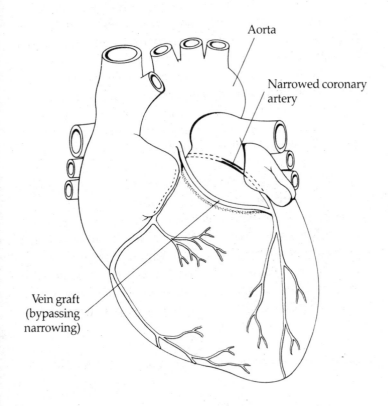

Figure 6   *Coronary artery bypass graft (CABG or Cabbage operation)*

often used in the diagnosis of angina, the assessment of need for surgery and the assessment of recovery after a heart attack.

Balloons and lasers

In early 1980 Dr David Cumberland, consultant radiologist at the Northern General Hospital, was the first doctor in the United Kingdom to use a very special balloon to dilate, or open up, the coronary arteries in patients suffering from severe coronary artery narrowing. This operation is now available at many of the cardiac centres throughout the world.

Dr Cumberland, who divides his working life between Sheffield and the San Francisco Heart Institute in California, has also pioneered even newer techniques which involve burning a clear passage through a completely blocked coronary artery either with a laser or with ultrasound waves emitted by a very fine probe. When you realize that these techniques are performed through a tiny puncture in the femoral artery at the top of the leg, so that all there is to see afterwards is some bruising, you will begin to appreciate just how wonderful this technology has become. The drawing (see *Figure 7*) shows how a balloon is used to dilate a narrowed coronary artery in the procedure which is called angio-plasty (angio = blood vessel, plasty = plastic modification).

Figure 7   *Using a balloon to open up a narrowed coronary artery*

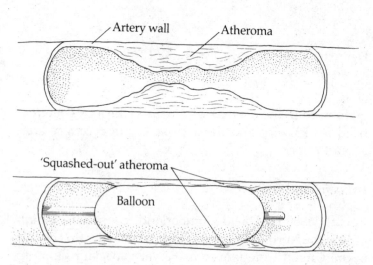

After the big 'H'

Everybody who has suffered a heart attack feels depressed about it. It's only natural to expect this – after all, a heart attack is a painful and frightening reminder of mortality. There is often something of an emotional crisis when the sufferer returns home, with feelings of inadequacy and the sense that life will never be the same again. For most people this need not be the case at all.

In fact most people make a good recovery after a heart attack and they can often return to all the activity they enjoyed before it. Heavy or very stressful work is probably not advisable, but even then some people do insist on returning to it and appear to cope very well.

One thing you need to avoid is the so-called 'cardiac neurosis', in which an individual cannot forget that he or she has had a heart attack and lives in such a state of anxiety that they imagine all sorts of things being the matter with them when in fact they have made a perfectly good recovery. Your doctor will advise you on how much activity you can return to. Remember that some heart attacks are so minor that people do not even know they have suffered them, while a small proportion may indeed be very severe. The severity depends on the amount of damaged muscle and, as advised earlier in the chapter, getting to hospital quickly may help to keep this to a minimum. Thrombolytic treatment and emergency angioplasty offer all sorts of possibilities for the future.

Immediately after leaving hospital, the sufferer should be given clear guidance on the gradual resumption of exercise. The aim is to resume normal life, and often the same type of work, about twelve weeks after the heart attack. This is not the place to give very detailed guidance – the best people to give you advice are the hospital staff and your family doctor, who will have the details of your case. Every person has his or her own heart attack, and the speed of recovery will be equally individual.

Do I need to change my way of life?

Quite possibly you do – not in some dreadful way that will make you a cardiac invalid, but in the more common sense way we advocate in this book. Often factors in your way of life will have led to the heart attack in the first place. Remember, this book is as much for somebody who has had a heart attack already as for somebody who has never had one – and wishes to do her or his utmost to avoid having one.

General guides to recovery

These are only broad guides, and your case may have special circumstances which require a different approach. If you feel anxious or depressed, the guide to relaxation in Chapter 10 might help you. Sleep may be a problem, but try not to get hooked on sleeping tablets, which are often very difficult to stop.

With exercise, gradually increase the amount you do. Restrict the number of times you climb the stairs for the first two weeks at home; after that you will probably find yourself back to normal in this respect. Walking is the most beneficial and simple exercise of all, but take it slowly. Avoid walking out after a heavy meal or in very cold weather. It is probably not wise to return to very competitive sports such as squash for a very long time. Within four weeks of going home you will be walking half a mile or so. Within eight weeks you should be able to walk a mile or so on the flat. But if it tires you or makes you breathless, slacken off and build up slowly again.

If you are overweight, then gradually get your weight down to the recommended normal for your height, sex and build. The low saturated fat diet recommended in this book will certainly help most people.

With diet in general, we recommend the Eskimo Diet to all after a heart attack, provided there are not exceptional factors such as an allergy to fish or other dietary recommendations made by a specialist such as the hospital dietician. For instance, a patient discovered to have severe cholesterol problems in the blood may have to take a therapeutic diet, sometimes coupled with medication. But for most people the diet recommended here is the ideal.

When can I have sex?

As a general rule we advise people to wait four to six weeks. This again will vary with the size of the heart attack. The guide should be that it does not provoke symptoms such as pain, breathlessness or exhaustion.

What about returning to work?

Somebody with a light and not too stressful job will often return to work early, say at about seven or eight weeks. Most will need to wait about twelve weeks. Try to make an arrangement with your boss to return to normal activity gradually. If you are worried about the heavy nature of the work or the effects of high pressure, take a good long think, discuss it with your spouse or friends, then go and talk to your boss, your personnel officer or your medical officer. If you are still uncertain, discuss it with your doctor and consider talking to your local Disablement Resettlement Office (DRO). The DRO will be contactable either through the hospital or at your local government employment agency. She or he specializes in linking medical difficulty or disability with appropriate employment and acts as a go-between between doctor and employer, very often much to your advantage.

What about driving?

If you are the holder of a heavy goods vehicle licence (HGV) or a public service vehicle licence (PSV) then, sadly, you will not be allowed to keep it after you have had a heart attack. It may surprise you to discover that anybody who has had a heart attack is required by law to report it to the DVLC at Swansea before resuming driving, and this applies even if you feel back to normal health. You must do this before you drive again, and not wait until the licence expires. In practice the vast majority of people who have had a heart attack will quickly return to social driving again, usually about two months after their return home. The DVLC might write, with your permission, either to your GP or the hospital specialist, but unless there are unusual circumstances, such as unpredictable blackouts, they will sanction your driving again.

Are there any do's and don'ts?

If you were a smoker, it is vital you give up smoking completely. Don't just reduce or switch to a pipe or cigars.

Don't allow yourself to fall into a well of depression and worry. Get back as closely as possible to normal life.

Read the advice sections of this book very carefully. Aim at an enthusiastic and enjoyable new life, with a healthy attitude to exercise, stress and happiness. Follow the Eskimo Diet described in detail in Chapter 8.

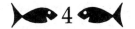

The Importance of Diet

There is an old joke in medical circles that if you put ten experts into a debate, you will get twenty opinions. One will declare that lowering cholesterol in the diet, for instance, will greatly reduce the risk of a heart attack, while another will insist that it won't make a jot of difference. This debate has raged for at least twenty-five years and the various arguments would fill ten books the size of this one. Why is there such confusion?

There is no doubt at all that if you have raised blood cholesterol, known medically as hyper-cholesterolaemia, you are running an increased risk of suffering a heart attack. The difficulty lies in proving that if doctors lower your blood cholesterol – which is usually quite easy to achieve by diet alone – this actually reduces your risk. Doubts have been expressed by the distinguished epidemiologist Professor A. G. Shaper at London University and the distinguished cardiologist Professor Michael F. Oliver at Edinburgh University. Another problem is that all the early medical studies looked at the total level of cholesterol in people's blood – but now we know that the blood contains different kinds of cholesterol. Finally, medical trials concerned with heart disease are much more difficult to conduct than trials dealing with other conditions.

If we doctors were attempting to heal duodenal ulcers,

for example, we could take a hundred patients, offer them two alternative treatments, and at the end of two months we could check how many ulcers had healed in each group. But when it comes to preventing heart attacks with diet, matters are much more complicated. We would have to set up a trial with large numbers of patients (hundreds or even thousands) over anything from two to twenty years – and to add to these difficulties we would have to show that something that might be expected to happen did not happen.

Doctors are also reluctant to recommend any treatment until it is definitely proven to work. If somebody is offered a treatment that has had exaggerated claims made for it, only to discover it does not work, the additional disappointment on top of the sad outcome is all the more unbearable for the patient and her or his family. Doctors are not unwilling to consider new treatments, but they must be sure that the treatments are safe and that they work.

Only rarely is a line of research so productive that nearly all the researchers concur. Compared to cholesterol research, the work done on the beneficial effects of fish oil has seen very little disagreement. A single review article published in 1988 in the prestigious *Journal of the American Medical Association* referred to 119 separate scientific studies of the properties of fish or fish oil, conducted in the most respected hospitals and university centres in the world and by the most eminent doctors and scientists – and almost every study pointed to some unusual and potentially beneficial effects. The story of this important advance in our knowledge will be described in Chapter 5.

But let's return meanwhile to the cholesterol controversy. If it has divided the medical world for a generation, how much more confusing it all must be to the public! So what *is* this fiendish public enemy number one?

What is cholesterol?

Cholesterol is found as a natural substance in all animal cells and blood. It is an essential element in our body chemistry – indeed we do not need to take it in our diets at all, because it is important enough for our bodies to produce it. In other words, it isn't a demon come to ravage mankind in the twentieth century. It is more a question of balance – and we have got the balance wrong.

Notwithstanding the conflicting opinions of the experts, an overall conclusion can be drawn from the mass of cholesterol research. In countries such as the UK, with a high average level of total blood cholesterol, the population runs a high risk of a heart attack.

Inherited raised blood cholesterol

Some people have what is called a familial tendency to high blood cholesterol – in other words it is an inherited problem. If several members of your family have suffered heart attacks (a history of sudden death is often very indicative), particularly in their forties, thirties or even younger, then you might be suffering from hereditary raised cholesterol. This affects about one person in five hundred and is referred to medically as hereditary or familial hypercholesterolaemia.

The risk of a heart attack for a patient with familial raised blood cholesterol is eight times the normal. If you suspect you may have inherited this problem, it is simple to arrange with your family doctor for the fat levels in your blood to be tested. A blood sample, taken when you are fasting, should include tests for cholesterol, HDL-cholesterol, triglyceride, and, hopefully, a calculation of the HDL/LDL-cholesterol ratio. Don't let the scientific terms put you off – they will all be explained a little later. The condition nearly always responds to dietary advice, although a few people may need to take a medication that lowers their cholesterol. Advice on this will be given by your family doctor – or in some cases by a hospital specialist if your doctor thinks it necessary.

Who should have their blood fats screened?

We make no apology for what may appear a controversial statement: everybody in the population should be screened. Yes, this does include children, especially if there is a strong family history of coronary heart disease or known high risk of atheroma. In families with hereditary high blood fats, even very young children may be affected and must be screened. All the big atheroma trials have indicated that it starts early in childhood, so the sooner we spot high-risk people and do something about it the better. Screening is possible on the Health Service or privately and it only involves a simple blood test.

What are HDL-cholesterol and LDL-cholesterol?

Cholesterol is manufactured mainly in our livers – and, as already noted, is a vital chemical for our body cells. How does it get to all of these cells, since it is completely insoluble in water?

The answer is that it has to be kept in solution by some tricky chemistry inside our vital organs. The body produces particles made up of protein and fat that act as transporters for cholesterol in our blood – in other words it is carried about dissolved in tiny little droplets. These transporting particles are recognized by receiving stations on the walls of our cells, where the cholesterol is accepted. The process continues in a businesslike manner – until something goes wrong.

The main particle involved in ferrying cholesterol is low density lipoprotein or LDL. It arrives at the liver, picks up its cargo of cholesterol, and transports it into the blood en route for the cells throughout the body. Problems arise if there are too few sites in the tissues for the LDL to dock at, and so it starts to dump its load in all sorts of areas where this really shouldn't happen. This is why doctors are more interested these days in a high level of LDL-cholesterol than in a high level of whole-blood cholesterol.

One of these unwelcome dumping grounds is the lining of the coronary arteries. Now the process of atheroma, explained in Chapter 2, can be fully understood. The frightening thing for us in the Western world is that this excessive dumping of fat, or atheroma, starts so early in life; the very first evidence of the process can be seen in the coronary arteries of young children. Pathologists who performed post-mortems on young American soldiers killed in the Korean War were astonished to find such advanced atheroma in men who were barely out of their teens.

Obviously, we in the Western world eat too much cholesterol and this adds to the body's problems of overloading. But the way to deal with this situation is not an obsessive preoccupation with every milligram of cholesterol in our diet. Indeed the problem has more to do with saturated fat than with cholesterol, and this will be explained a little later.

There is an ancient theory called the Doctrine of Agues, which says that wherever you find a malady, a benevolent providence will have also provided the cure. All you have to do is look for it. In the human body, providence has provided a counter to excess cholesterol in another small particle called high density lipoprotein, or HDL. This, too, is produced in the liver. As the HDL circulates, its main function is to scavenge excess tissue cholesterol, which it picks up and returns to the liver for disposal.

An eminent doctor in the United States, William Castelli, reported that a man in his early thirties had died in his sleep; the results of a post-mortem examination showed that his arteries were hopelessly furred up with cholesterol-laden atheroma. The baffling thing was that this unfortunate man did not have high blood cholesterol. Intrigued, Dr Castelli investigated more closely.

He discovered that the young man's ability to clear cholesterol from the blood was very poor. So although his total cholesterol was normal, he could not ferry it properly into the receiving stations in the tissues. He had a low blood HDL. Subsequent research has confirmed this finding. If you have a low HDL-cholesterol you are at greater risk of a heart attack.

Your total cholesterol/HDL-cholesterol ratio

A quick way to find out if you have a high risk factor for heart attacks is, once you have had your blood fats tested, to divide your HDL-cholesterol count into your total cholesterol count. If the figure you get is around 4.95, you have an average risk. If the figure is higher than this your risk increases, and if it is lower the risk is less than average.

Dietary advice is dealt with fully in Chapter 8. Meanwhile, here is an interesting fact: adding oily fish or pure fish oil to your diet can increase your level of protective HDL-cholesterol. Your body does this by modifying the chemistry of another fat called triglyceride.

What are triglycerides?

Examples are the white 'lardy' fat you see on meat, on the top of a pint of fresh full-cream milk, or floating in the pan as all-too-delicious melting butter! This is the kind of fat that contains those well-known risk factors referred to as *saturates* and *unsaturates*, which will be explained below.

Triglycerides are made up of two main ingredients. The first of these is called glycerol, and a single molecule of glycerol has the chemical shape of a three-pronged gardening fork. The second ingredient, called fatty acids, comes in three parcels, each of which bonds itself to one prong of the glycerol molecule. This new chemical, made from the joining of three molecules of fatty acid on to one molecule of glycerol, is called a triglyceride.

As fats, triglycerides are one of the body's most important energy sources. Gram for gram, they are more energy-rich than sugar or carbohydrate. They can be taken directly from the food we eat or can be manufactured in the liver, where they are used to store energy for when we make our muscles work hard and require a large supply of triglycerides.

Why is triglyceride so important in preventing heart attacks? When Hugh Sinclair examined Eskimos in their natural environment he found that, although they were virtually free of heart attacks, their blood cholesterol level was quite close to that in the United Kingdom. What was different was the level of their triglyceride. In spite of their very high intake of animal fat, the level of their triglyceride was only a quarter of the average level in the UK.

Here in the Western world, if we eat a lot of fat we can expect high triglyceride levels in our blood. The early pioneers such as Sinclair expected high levels in Eskimos and were astonished to find that the triglyceride levels were so very low in their blood. At the time they were utterly baffled. We believe we now know the explanation: there are fatty acids unique to fish which actually lower triglyceride in our blood. We shall return to this topic shortly.

General advice about being overweight

What we mean when we talk about unwanted body fat is stored triglyceride. When we eat this kind of fat it is broken down in the gut by digestive enzymes, only to be reassembled within the body and transported by another of the protein carrier molecules, VLDL (very low density lipoprotein), to our fat stores, where it usually makes us unhappy. In women fat is preferentially distributed to the bust, bottom, abdomen and thighs. In men it shows a more even body distribution, although they too show a marked tendency to accumulate it in the big elastic space between the chest and the pelvis.

The more we eat of foods containing triglyceride, the more fat is stored: it is, more or less, a simple equation. Fat is energy stored. When we exercise, whether it be a gentle walk or a tough game of football or hockey, our muscles need a supply of energy. The body nips off a bit of fat from our reserves and chops down the molecule so that the fatty acids (now called free fatty acids) are released, to be burnt up in the muscle cells. If we do no more exercise than walking to the television set or the biscuit box then we won't burn up a great deal of fat. Unfortunately there is a vicious circle in which we continue to eat food at a rate laid down in our more energetic youth, fat builds up in those bulgy bits of us, we get slower and feel less like exercising, and so on.

Being fat does not itself lead directly to a heart attack, although it is linked closely with several factors that do increase the risk, such as hypertension, raised blood triglyceride levels, raised blood cholesterol levels and reduced physical activity. If these other factors are not present, then, surprisingly, obesity in itself is not a risk factor. Even more surprising, perhaps, is the fact that those people who can binge on food to their heart's desire and still remain reed-slim are not immune to heart attacks.

How does this relate to heart attacks?

Our researches have shown that in people with a higher than normal triglyceride level, tested while they are fasting, the HDL is usually lower than it should be. If we reduce our blood triglyceride by cutting down on saturated fat in our food, the HDL in our blood will probably increase. Here we encounter another of those wonderful properties of fish oil. Although it is a fatty acid, it has powerful protective effects on the level of triglyceride in our blood.

Alcohol and sugar

Sadly, alcohol does have the effect of raising fat levels in the blood; and so, if indulged to excess, does sugar. But don't get depressed – it's all a matter of balance and common sense. We would not claim conclusive proof that a glass of wine or beer a day actually helps – although the incidence of coronary heart disease is a lot lower in France than in the United Kingdom – but, taken in moderate quantities, alcohol increases our enjoyment of life and certainly does not cause the vast majority of the population any harm. Nor do we say you cannot have any butter, cheese, meat, milk or sugar. What we are saying is that in the United Kingdom we consume *too much* of these products.

Oral contraceptives

Some pills increase cholesterol and triglyceride, while others are actually beneficial, increasing HDL-cholesterol. In general it appears to be the oestrogen in the pill which is beneficial to women, and the newer pills have been formulated with this, amongst many other factors, in mind.

Exercise

Other activities to increase the protective levels of HDL in our blood include exercise, weight reduction, and in general a healthier, fitter lifestyle.

What are fatty acids?

Let's talk just a little about another of those components that make up the complete molecule of triglyceride – the fatty acids.

These are the 'polywhatsits' that give the Sunday newspapers such fun in their headline material. They are the basic components of all fats and oils – indeed they are the building blocks from which fats and oils are made. There are three common types of fatty acids, saturated, polyunsaturated and monounsaturated. The physical differences between these three types may appear to be trivial, but in the internal chemistry of our bodies such differences are devastatingly vital.

Saturated fats

A fatty acid is basically like an open necklace of carbon atoms (like little black pearls) with an acid chemical

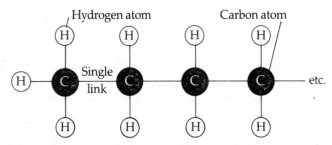

Notice all links between carbons are single, this allows
every carbon 2 or 3 hydrogen links, hence 'hydrogenated'

Figure 8   *A saturated fatty acid*

group at one end of it. If the chemical links between the
carbon pearls are single, the fat is saturated (see *Figure 8*).

Unsaturated fats

If any of the links are double, the fat is unsaturated. One
double link (called a chemical double bond) and it's a
monounsaturate. Two or more along the necklace (chemical chain) and it's a *polyunsaturated* fatty acid.

Hydrogenated fats

Saturated is a chemical term referring to whether or not
you can attach any more hydrogen atoms. If there are
no double links left, you cannot. If there are, you can
break a double link into a single, releasing two more
chemical positions to which hydrogen atoms can be
attached. This also explains another confusing term,
hydrogenated, which is frequently found in nutritional
labels on food. For example, a hydrogenated vegetable
oil may have started out life as a polyunsaturate, but
hydrogenation means the double links have been broken
and hydrogen added. The vegetable oil is therefore no
longer a polyunsaturate but a saturate.

Examples of saturated and unsaturated fats

One or two examples will put you in the picture. Lard or dripping is composed mainly of saturated fatty acids (the ones that are bad for us) and this results in a hard fat. Olive oil is composed mainly of monounsaturated fatty acids and is quite fluid in warm temperatures, but can become thick and less runny when cold. Corn and vegetable oils are mostly polyunsaturated fatty acids and remain fluid at quite low temperatures. All these are listed and described in Chapter 8.

Saturated fats are nothing other than fats that contain mostly saturated fatty acids, whether in their native chemical state or making up part of triglyceride molecules. For many years we have indulged ourselves in large quantities of saturated fats in the form of chips, Sunday joints and roast potatoes cooked in the meat dripping, not to mention the tasty traditional bacon, eggs, fried bread and, in Northern England, Scotland and Ireland, black and white puddings, which are enormously high in saturated fat. If you knew how much saturated fat beef and pork sausages contain, you would be very surprised!

Why saturated fat is bad for modern man

This story can be used to sum up the effects and functions of blood fats. It is set in a forest in Ancient Britain. A young man, entirely naked except for a coat of blue woad (or was it the British climate?), was squatting and eating his lunch while looking furtively over one shoulder and then the other. No doubt he was afraid of being attacked by a sabre-toothed tiger or some such hungry animal. Suddenly there was a roar behind him and immediately his heart started to race as the adrenalin flowed. At the same time triglyceride was released from his fat stores and converted into free fatty acids to supply energy for his escape. He ran and ran until he could no longer hear his enemy behind him; in so doing he used up the released triglyceride and his heart slowed down as the adrenalin supply decreased. As well as increasing the heart rate, adrenalin also increases blood triglyceride levels.

His modern counterpart is likely to be sitting in his office when the telephone rings. His boss exclaims, 'What the hell happened to that report I asked for – do something about it!' Immediately our poor friend's adrenalin flows, his heart rate goes up and his triglyceride level is raised. But does he immediately spring into all-out exercise to use up this potential energy? He is far more likely to tense up over his desk, light a cigarette and stew in his high adrenalin, persistently raised triglyceride, ongoing high heart rate and raised blood pressure.

To give another example, closer to our own times, people will often point to one of their elderly relatives and say: 'But look at my grandmother! She's eaten dripping and cream all her life and she's ninety-two.' This may well be true. But the grandmother in question usually worked very hard physically in the home, did not have a car to ferry her to work or to the shops, never sat back for hours watching television, did not live and work in a centrally heated environment, and so on. There is a balance between fat consumed and energy output, and today we exercise a great deal less than our parents and grandparents.

So what is special about fish?

Imagine what would happen if fish, living in cold waters, were fed the saturated fats we tend to eat! The cold would make the fats in their blood congeal, and the

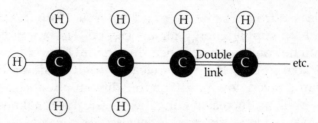

Notice the double link (chemical 'double band') at the
'3' carbon position. For carbons '3' and '4' there is only
1 available link for hydrogen

Figure 9   *An Omega-3 (or n-3) unsaturated fatty acid*

blood flow would slow down until the fish became as
stiff as a board. Clearly they must eat polyunsaturates
of a special kind which remain fluid at cold temperatures.

Fish contain special fats because they themselves eat
polyunsaturated fats of a very special type. These fats
have a double link between the third and fourth carbon
pearl, the so-called '3' position, and so they are called
n-3 (or Omega 3) fatty acids (see *Figure 9*).

The vital Omega-3 fatty acids in fish oil

The vital ingredients in fish oil, EPA and DHA, which
are much easier to remember than what they stand for,
the tongue-twisting eicosapentanoic acid and docosa-
hexaenoic acid, are two of those n-3 polyunsaturated
fatty acids. But they are very special ones, known as
'essential' fatty acids. Indeed your body cannot make
them on its own (no more than the fish can – they eat
it in plankton), so the only way you can get them into
your cells is by eating them in your diet. And the only
food that contains these very special ingredients in any
significant quantity is oily fish. If EPA and DHA are only
found in oily fish, what will be the consequences of not
eating fish as part of our normal diet?

5

The Scientific Evidence

Science has often been tagged with the labels 'mad' and 'bad', like Dr Strangelove, whereas in reality it comprises a lifetime of hard, repetitive work, often with temporary setbacks and disappointments. Only rarely does an avenue of research prove as fruitful as the fish oil story. After Hugh Sinclair's pioneering start with the Eskimos, you can imagine the scepticism of the medical world – a feeling that remains prevalent today. The view was well summed up by Dr Jack Yetiv in a paper published in 1988 in the *Journal of the American Medical Association*, which we shall discuss in more detail later in this chapter: 'While physicians tend to avoid items sold in health food stores, they eagerly embrace products of pharmaceutical laboratories. Although avoidance of most popular remedies is usually scientifically support-able, this appears not to be the case with fish oils, or their active ingredients, n-3 fatty acids.'

Of course some degree of scepticism is necessary in science. But what Dr Yetiv is suggesting is that doctors may be unduly sceptical of fish oil because it seems so ordinary (even doctors' mothers doled out cod liver oil to their children). The medical profession is a little reluc-tant to believe that something available over the counter in the chemist's shop could have such breakthrough importance in heart attacks. This point is a very important one, and it can only be answered by hard scientific evidence.

The two Danish scientists, Jorn Dyerberg and Hans Bang, who accompanied Hugh Sinclair on his journey to Greenland in 1976 took samples of Eskimo blood back with them to the hospital in Denmark where they worked. When they analysed the fats in this blood, what they found surprised them greatly. In addition to the low blood triglyceride and other changes in such important components as HDL-cholesterol, they discovered profound differences in the presence of those essential fatty acids EPA and DHA.

Dyerberg and Bang found that these were plentiful in the blood and tissue of Eskimos, while they were hardly present at all in the blood of people who ate a Western diet – and the degree of difference was enormous. Of course we now know that, if you don't eat fish or take fish oil, the levels in your body will be zero.

The sixty-four thousand dollar question must be quite obvious. What do these fatty acids do in our bodies? Do they play any important part in our internal chemistry? If they do, our chemistry would obviously be disturbed if they were missing.

Much of the scientific evidence has been published in the medical press. It would be unreasonable to expect you to take what we say at its face value without further supporting testimony from other doctors and scientists. We shall therefore be quoting from a number of scientific papers in this chapter, but without confusing the issue by using obscure jargon and medical terminology.

For those of our readers with a medical or scientific background we have included a small number of journal references, because these papers would provide a trained person with convenient starting points for information.

The four key papers

These papers are what is known as review papers – detailed, impartial summaries of all the research done to date on an important subject, written by a very experienced expert at the forefront of that research.

Author: Clemens von Shacky, Division of Hematology/ Oncology, New York Veterans' Administration Medical Center and Cornell University Medical College, New York. Title: *Prophylaxis of Atherosclerosis with Marine Omega-3 Fatty Acids. A Comprehensive Strategy.* Published in *Annals of Internal Medicine,* 1987, volume 107, pages 890–9.

Authors: Alexander Leaf and Peter C. Weber, Department of Preventive Medicine and Clinical Epidemiology, Harvard Medical School, Boston, and the Institut für Prophylaxe und Epidemiologie der Kreislaufkrankheiten, Universität München, Munich. Title: *Cardiovascular Effects of n-3 Fatty Acids.* Published in *New England Journal of Medicine,* 1988, volume 318, pages 549–57.

Author: T. A. B. Sanders, Department of Food and Nutritional Sciences, King's College, University of London. Title: *Fish and Coronary Artery Disease.* Published in *British Heart Journal,* 1987, volume 57, pages 214–19.

Author: Jack Zeev Yetiv, Department of Emergency Medicine, Sequoia Hospital, Redwood City, California. Title: *Clinical Applications of Fish Oils.* Published in *Journal of the American Medical Association,* 1988, volume 260, pages 665–70.

These four papers will be quoted from as appropriate in this chapter. They will be referred to simply by the surname of their author or authors.

What happens to the fat levels in our blood when we eat fish or take fish oil?

First of all the triglyceride level falls dramatically. Dr Saynor has published several careful studies on this effect, confirmed by other research workers throughout the world.

After a fatty meal this level normally shoots up, but after taking fish oil even the rise in blood levels after such a meal is dramatically reduced. Dr Saynor has also shown that this is usually accompanied by a significant rise in the protective HDL-cholesterol and by a smaller fall in the total blood cholesterol. Occasional reports have questioned the cholesterol effects, but Yetiv is quite convincing in his summing-up of this evidence.

Leaf and Weber, in their comprehensive review, draw attention to this powerful effect in reducing not only triglyceride but one of the most dangerous forms of blood fats, VLDL. Fish oil lowers both these types of fat in the blood – and not only in people with high blood fat levels to start with. 'In subjects with normal levels of triglycerides, considerably smaller amounts [of fish or oil] will lower these concentrations.' Fish oil has a much smaller effect on high blood cholesterol levels in those people with an inherited tendency, although the protective HDL-cholesterol is often increased.

Does improvement in blood fats have any beneficial effects on the formation of atheroma?

Animal experimentation excites ethical and emotional debate, but undoubtedly some useful medical information is obtained from it. Studies with animals have repeatedly demonstrated the protective value of fish oils in preventing atheroma. Dr R. W. Landymore of Dalhousie University, Canada, looked at the ability of fish oil to prevent the thickening of the lining of grafts such as are used in coronary artery bypass operations. He and his colleagues tested dogs by giving one group a high-cholesterol diet and another group the same diet but with additional cod liver oil. When these two groups were given experimental vein grafts, the dogs on the high-cholesterol diet very quickly developed atheroma in their grafts. The dogs given an identical diet (who developed similarly high blood cholesterol levels) developed hardly any signs of atheroma in their grafts. In another study, these same researchers compared the effects of aspirin and persantin (conventional medical therapy) to that of fish oil in preventing atheromatous change in grafts, and found that fish oil was better.

Dr B. H. Weiner and colleagues from the University of Massachusetts looked at the effects of cod liver oil in pigs which were fed a diet of saturated fats and cholesterol that gave them high levels of blood cholesterol. As with the dogs, one group was also given fish oil. After eight months the coronary arteries of the pigs not given oil were markedly furred up, whereas those given fish oil had significantly less development of atheroma. Interestingly, this protective quality of fish oil occurred when the cholesterol of the oil-fed group of pigs was still very high.

Other researchers have shown the same protection against atheromatous hardening of the arteries in rhesus monkeys and in rabbits. Although animals are clearly different in many respects from humans, in fact these animal experiments conform very closely with the observed effects of fish oil in humans. Two very recent reports illustrate this very interesting potential in humans.

At Toyama Medical University, Japan, Dr T. Hamazaki and colleagues compared the thickening of the great artery, the aorta, between the inhabitants of two Japanese villages. One group lived by fishing and had a high intake of fish in their diet, while the other was a farming village, where they ate much less fish. The researchers found that the high fish eaters had significantly less hardening of the artery than the low fish eaters.

At the Department of Medicine and Surgery, Monash University, Melbourne, Dr M. L. Wahlqvist studied the artery walls of both healthy people and a group of long-standing diabetic patients. Diabetic patients were chosen because this condition is associated with an increased incidence of atheroma. When the researchers compared fish eaters and non-fish eaters in their two groups, they found significantly greater hardening of the arteries in the non-fish eaters. This was most significant in the so-called 'healthy' group.

A number of other studies by researchers such as Drs D. H. Blankenhorn, R. Brandt and their colleagues at the University of Southern California have demonstrated the possibility that atheroma in human beings can be not only halted but even reversed with therapy that lowers blood fats. Further research needs to be done to confirm their findings and produce a detailed evaluation.

What happens to the clotting tendency in our blood when we eat fish or take fish oil?

We were recently asked a very important question indeed. If most of us already have narrowed arteries, or atheroma – as we unfortunately do – is there any use in following the Eskimo Diet? The answer, most positively, is: Yes!

Remember that second vital part of the equation that causes a heart attack: the clot of blood within the already narrowed artery. Although we have narrowed arteries, the vast majority of us feel perfectly well and can get about, perform our jobs and enjoy life to the full. So if we can prevent that clot forming (and all the more so if we can halt, perhaps even improve, the furring up process in the arteries) we would do ourselves a power of good. Consider what is known about the causes of the clot itself.

Platelet stickiness

The stickiness of the platelets, the little gum-like bodies in our blood, is very important. The platelet actually contains fatty acid as part of its normal composition, and the type of fatty acid our platelets contain depends precisely on what enters our bodies through our diet.

The normal sort of fatty acid present in platelets (n-6) tends to promote the release of a clotting substance whose scientific name is thromboxane A2. This makes the platelets very sticky and more liable to form a blood clot. Taking fish or fish oil means that a different fatty acid enters our platelets, the n-3 fatty acid called EPA. This has a dramatic effect, causing another type of clotting substance called thromboxane A3 to be formed by the platelet.

It is very easy to get confused between such similar-sounding chemical substances as A2 and A3, but they have markedly different effects on our body chemistry. A large number of studies worldwide have demonstrated this effect of fish oil. The A3 thromboxane tends to do the opposite of the A2: it prevents the platelets becoming excessively sticky. This, as you might imagine, reduces the blood's tendency to form dangerous clots.

Taking fish or fish oil in reasonable amounts does not, of course, stop platelets from clotting altogether; if it did, we would bleed to death from a minor cut. What it appears to do is to reduce the likelihood of clotting within arteries while retaining the normal pattern of protection against bleeding.

Aspirin treatment

This platelet stickiness factor is the basis for the use of aspirin as a preventive treatment for heart attacks and strokes. Many very good studies have confirmed this role for aspirin. Isn't it a little ironical that here we have another beneficial treatment that our mothers and grandmothers believed in? Simple aspirin, taken in a small dose – one tablet every day, or every second day – reduces platelet stickiness, and in large studies it has been shown to reduce the risk of a second heart attack in people who have already suffered one. Aspirin is indeed very safe overall, but in a minority of people it causes bleeding from the stomach – it is therefore usually avoided by people with a known history of peptic ulcers. There is now an abundance of evidence that fish oil has a similar effect on platelet stickiness to aspirin.

Leaf and Weber conclude:

It should be noted that aspirin, which is widely used to prevent coronary artery disease, is prescribed only to block the platelet production of thromboxane [the A2 variety described above] whereas n-3 fatty acids interfere with the pathophysiologic developments in atherosclerosis at several loci. Thus, n-3 fatty acids may have more clinical benefits than aspirin, even though aspirin is a more effective inhibitor of thromboxane synthesis.

In other words, aspirin is slightly better at this effect on platelets, but fish oil does have the same sort of effect plus the bonus of all sorts of other benefits that aspirin does not possess.

A few words of caution: if you are taking aspirin on your doctor's advice, don't take it into your own head to change things. Some doctors worry that because aspirin and fish oil have similar effects on platelets they should not be taken together. In fact, as part of Dr Saynor's heart attack study a number of patients took aspirin as well as quite large doses of fish oil – some even took anticoagulants (blood thinners) as well – and there were no bleeding complications. However, such studies were conducted within the safety of a hospital, where repeated checks of blood function were easily possible.

While we believe that, in the small and natural doses we recommend for general use, it is almost certainly safe to add fish oil to the small doses of aspirin (usually one tiny tablet a day) that are conventionally taken to prevent heart attacks, this may not apply to people taking larger doses for conditions such as severe arthritis. Like many other ingredients in our diet, such as alcohol, salt, fat and sugar, it is a question of getting the balance right. Quantity is very important. If you are taking more than one aspirin tablet a day or if you are on anticoagulant drugs such as warfarin, fish oil should only be taken under medical supervision. The large doses of fish oil that have been prescribed in certain controlled medical trials are a different matter entirely, and once again should only be taken under medical supervision.

The blood-clotting protein, fibrinogen

The platelet clot is reinforced by a much more permanent blood clot in our bloodstream, caused by the clotting factors in our blood. A vital component in forming this permanent clot is the protein called fibrinogen. Several studies have shown that the fibrinogen level tends to be high in people who have suffered a heart attack. Smoking is one of the factors that raise fibrinogen. Studies by Dr Saynor, confirmed in several other medical centres, show that fish oil reduces blood fibrinogen levels, making it less likely to form dangerous clots.

Blood viscosity

But there are many more properties of fish oils that help to prevent clots. For example, if the flow is thicker (increased viscosity), the blood is more liable to clot. Fish oil reduces the viscosity so that the blood will flow more freely in all our arteries – yet another beneficial effect on a known risk factor for heart attacks. This is partly due to an important change in our red blood cells.

Red blood cells

Our red cells are very pliable, and loss of pliability is believed to be another important factor in heart attacks. Red cells need to be able to change their shape in order to pass down fine arteries – remember some arteries are as small as 1/16 inch. Our red blood cells are sometimes three times the diameter of the little blood vessels they have to squeeze through, but the body enables the cells to go on their way by making the membrane covering the red cell elastic and supple. However, in some people who are prone to heart attacks, particularly if they eat a lot of saturated fat, the pliability of their red blood cells is reduced. This makes the blood flow to vital organs such as the heart and brain dwindle. When EPA and DHA fatty acids, which enter our bodies only from eating fish or taking fish oil, become incorporated into the red cell membrane they make the cell more pliable and able to squeeze through those narrow arteries.

The message is abundantly clear that eating fish or taking fish oil appears to affect, in a unique and very beneficial manner, the pathological processes that lead to a heart attack. But here we really must don our cynical hats and state that no amount of background research is enough – the arguments over cholesterol research have told us that. Research may suggest, but will never prove, that if you give fish or fish oil to real human beings with real diseases the stuff will actually work.

A true case history

One of Reg Saynor's patients, Bob, had a responsible job, and at the end of a day's work he liked nothing better than to come home and eat a good cooked dinner. He was especially fond of roast beef, Yorkshire pudding, roast potatoes (cooked in the juices – translate as saturated fats – of the meat) and all the trimmings. After a really good feed Bob would switch on the television, light his pipe and puff away contentedly, especially if football was on the box. As he got a little older (he was now fifty-two), he noticed a strange tingling sensation in his legs when he smoked his pipe in the evening. His wife persuaded him to visit his doctor, who arranged for him to have tests at the local hospital. Bob was shocked to be told that he had 'peripheral vascular disease', in other words that the arteries to his legs were furred up and narrowed. He was much relieved to notice a marked improvement when he threw his pipe into the dustbin. So what on earth happened to Bob?

Really it amounts to a combination of changes. First, the high saturated fat content of his food had produced a high fat level in his blood, making the blood more viscous and sluggish and more prone to form clots. The smoking aggravated this condition, and at the same time stimulated chemical changes which caused spasm in the arteries of his legs. Add to this the fact that years of the same eating and smoking pattern had already furred up his arteries, restricting the blood supply to his legs. The reason he improved when he stopped smoking was that one of the danger factors had been eliminated. With the Eskimo Diet a lot more could have been achieved – and he could still have had his favourite meal, though without the Yorkshire pudding and probably less often!

What happens when we give fish or fish oil to real people with real medical problems?

High blood pressure (hypertension)

Although the results of long-term trials with large numbers of patients have not yet been reported, in short-term trials fish oil has been shown to produce an improvement in people who were suffering from high blood pressure. The way in which fish oil achieves this is still under study. We mention this merely as yet another point of interest, and don't suggest that fish or fish oil should be taken as treatment for hypertension. The studies performed so far have been in patients taking high doses of fish oil or large amounts of fish daily, and would not correspond with the small doses we recommend. If you suffer from raised blood pressure, it is essential to go to your doctor for regular checks and to take whatever medication is prescribed.

Brain development

There is a good deal of evidence that the essential fatty acids in fish oil are necessary for brain development. Professor Crawford, head of nutritional biochemistry at the Nuffield Institute of Comparative Medicine, has reported on the importance of fish in our diet for the development and nutrition of our brains. He gives his evidence for this in a book called *The Driving Force*, published in 1989.

In 1982 an American doctor reported the case of a six-year-old girl who had been shot in the stomach, so that she had to be fed through a drip instead of eating food in the normal way. The drip fluid contained a lot of plant-derived n-6 fatty acids (the sort we take as vegetable oils), but little or no n-3 fish oil type of fatty acids. The child suffered visual and brain disturbances, but fortunately these disappeared rapidly when the doctors realized the nature of the problem and gave her a different fluid preparation containing n-3 fatty acids.

This case led a Scandanavian researcher to study a number of patients who had been in hospital for many years as a result of severe brain damage. Because they had been unable to feed themselves, they had had to be fed through a tube passed down the nose and into the stomach. They were found to have skin complaints and weight deficiencies which were corrected when n-3 fatty acids, previously missing, were added to the tube feeds.

Anti-inflammatory role

Many properly conducted scientific studies worldwide have demonstrated the benefits of taking fish oil for arthritis, the skin complaint called psoriasis, and several other medical conditions. At present research is just beginning on the investigation of a possible role for fish oil in treating the serious bowel condition known as ulcerative colitis, and many other studies are under way. It is now generally accepted by medical researchers that fish oil has unusual and very interesting anti-inflammatory properties, which are believed to be due to an alteration in the body's chemistry brought about by the unique fatty acids EPA and DHA.

Cancer

There is even a suggestion, though no conclusive scientific proof, that a diet high in saturated fat is linked to cancer of the breast and colon in humans, implying that a change of diet might reduce the risk.

Angina

This troublesome medical complaint, described in Chapter 2, is usually due to narrowing of the coronary arteries as a result of atheroma, but it can be caused by spasm in the coronary arteries and may be worsened by increased blood viscosity. In a large trial involving 107 people suffering from angina and reported in the journal *Atherosclerosis* in 1984, Dr Saynor found a marked improvement in their angina over a nine-month treatment period. Improvement was shown by dramatic reduction in the need to take glyceryl trinitrate tablets. This improvement could have resulted from changes in blood viscosity or from a reduced tendency of the platelets to clump, which again slows the blood circulating in the coronary arteries.

Dietary fish in the prevention of heart attacks

This is the most important of all the scientific evidence presented in this book. We shall look in a common-sense way at every known large-scale study that has examined the influence of eating fish on the rate of occurrence of heart attacks. The first was by Dr Avery M. Nelson, an American from Seattle, and was reported as long ago as 1972 in the journal *Geriatrics*.

The Nelson study

This study involved 206 patients under the age of seventy-five. Two-thirds had been referred to Dr Nelson because of high blood cholesterol and symptoms such as angina. Eighty patients were treated with a special diet, while another 126 acted as 'controls' and did not diet. As part of this special dietary assessment, Nelson tested the effects of seafood containing what he termed C22 fatty acids (nowadays we would assume that these also contained C20 fatty acids and were no different from what we call Omega-3 or n-3 fatty acids). Dr Nelson found that these high-risk patients survived much longer if they ate a diet rich in seafood. He concluded: 'Results from this study show that diets, including seafoods containing large amounts of Carbon 22 six double bond fatty acids, can be of considerable value in the treatment of patients with coronary problems.'

The Kromhout study

Kromhout and his colleagues got the idea for this study from the earlier reports of Sinclair, Dyerberg and Bang into the low death rate from heart attack amongst the Greenland Eskimos. Their subsequent work has been regarded as a milestone in the medical literature on fish and coronary heart disease.

The study was performed on 852 middle-aged men in the Dutch town of Zutphen, and was reported in the *New England Journal of Medicine* in 1985. Careful information about fish consumption in their diet was obtained from these men in 1960, when none of them had any symptoms or history of coronary disease. During twenty years of follow-up, seventy-eight of these men died from coronary disease.

This study clearly showed that men who ate fish had a significantly lower risk of dying from a heart attack. The authors tested their results vigorously with complicated statistical analyses to see of they could disprove this beneficial effect of fish, but they could not shake its validity. They declared: 'We conclude that the consumption of as little as one or two fish dishes per week may be of preventive value in relation to coronary heart disease.'

This was a faultlessly conducted scientific study, and it was the first to draw attention to the benefit of small 'doses' of fish. When Kromhout's paper was published it was immediately greeted with huge interest and not a little excitement. The editor of the *New England Journal* was soon flooded with letters from other doctors and medical scientists, giving their views and sometimes their own experiences of fish and coronary heart disease. Since these researchers' findings, unlike Kromhout's, were peripheral to the main aim of their respective studies, they must be treated with some caution.

The Shekelle study

Dr Richard B. Shekelle from the University of Texas, with the support of Dr Paul Oglesby from Harvard Medical School and others, was the author of one of these letters, published in the *New England Journal* in September 1985. Shekelle and his colleagues had published a formal study of the relationship between diet, blood cholesterol and death from coronary heart disease under the title 'Western Electric Study' in the same journal in 1981. They had included fish in their dietary questionnaire as part of that work, so now they could look specifically at fish consumption in their study group of approximately two thousand patients. Like Kromhout they had been studying middle-aged men, all of whom were free of coronary heart disease at the start of the study. These researchers now agreed with him that eating fish was associated with a reduced death rate from coronary heart disease.

Two other letters, however, did not agree with Kromhout. In fairness, and particularly since they are frequently referred to in medical articles, we should discuss these also.

The Vollset study

Dr Stein E. Vollset, of the University of Bergen, wrote a letter about an ongoing study that he and his colleagues were performing in Norway. They were investigating the links between diet and death from various types of diseases in seventeen thousand respondents to a postal survey of dietary habits. Their patients were nearly all fish eaters, so that a proper comparison between fish eaters and non-fish eaters was very difficult to make; if this study had been set up to test the fish hypothesis, the authors would have deliberately selected about equal numbers of fish eaters and non-fish eaters. The patients were also older on average at the start of the study than either Kromhout's or Shekelle's. The responses in 1967 to three questions on fish intake in their questionnaire formed the basis of a 'fish index', approximating the number of times fish was eaten per month. Their results appeared to show no tendency to fewer than expected fatal heart attacks among the high fish eaters.

Clearly this simple report should be regarded somewhat differently from Kromhout's carefully formulated, specifically focused study. There were additional problems in the Norwegian research, admitted by the authors, since not only was the study not designed from the outset to test the fish and heart attack hypothesis, but it was not even specifically orientated to assess new occurrences of heart attacks. As a result of this most of the men who died from coronary heart disease already had the disease at the start of the study. Only seventeen of the total of 967 deaths in patients with coronary heart disease were in men who had been free of disease to start with and who reported a level of fish consumption close to what we, in the United Kingdom, would class as average.

We do not mean to criticize the competence of the authors, who would not claim their letter as a formal study into the relationship between fish eating and heart attacks. The letter to the journal was just that, a letter, intended merely to give an indication of their experience gleaned from a study set up for other purposes. But even taking into account these serious limitations, there was a trend in the men under forty-five at the start of the study for fish intake to be associated with a reduced risk of death from coronary heart disease.

The Curb study

Once again this was a letter to the *New England Journal* rather than a formal study that answered a pre-set hypothesis. Dr J. David Curb and his colleague, Dwayne M. Reed, responded to Kromhout's study by retrospectively analysing previously recorded data from their Honolulu Heart Program. Since it was not primarily set up to test the fish and coronary heart disease relationship, we must be cautious in attributing too great a significance to the findings.

At the start of their twelve-year follow-up investigation of 7615 Japanese men, two kinds of information were obtained to determine fish consumption: the frequency of eating fish, and the amount of fish consumed during the previous twenty-four hours. The subjects of the study were nearly all fish eaters – only thirty-two men of a total of 7615 were non-fish eaters. The authors themselves drew attention to the small numbers of 'almost never' fish eaters and suggested that this should be taken into account when interpreting these data. Comparisons could only be made between people who ate fish less than twice a week and almost daily; even here there was a tendency for the high fish eaters to die less frequently from coronary heart disease, but it did not reach statistical significance.

Excitement and controversy

After the publication of Kromhout's results, which confirmed Dr Nelson's earlier report – and also given the intense background research which had gone on for almost a decade and pointed very strongly to an expected benefit from fish and fish oil – the US media and public were gripped by what might be termed 'Omega-3 fever'. A number of books were published, some good and others making rather extravagant claims given that the research was still in its preliminary stages at this time. The American medical establishment began to worry, particularly at the possibility that the public might be tempted to take big doses of fish oil in the belief that what was good for you in small amounts was sure to be even better for you in large amounts. Senior figures in the medical establishment warned the public to wait and see. We believe they were absolutely correct. A number of very important aspects were as yet to be explored.

Playing devil's advocate

Almost all the scientific evidence given above appears strongly to favour fish or fish oil. But is there any evidence *against* fish oil?

In fact the case against is so poor that we must look more to potential disadvantage than to anything that has been proven in forty years of intensive investigation in laboratories throughout the world. The safety aspects of fish oil will be discussed in detail at the end of Chapter 7. First, to test our own hypothesis, we should answer three vital questions.

Out of the many hundreds of studies, two raised an important query. These, by Peter Singer and colleagues in *Atherosclerosis* in 1986 and by Gordon Schectman and colleagues in *Annals of Internal Medicine* in 1989, enquired whether the effects of fish oil in lowering blood fats wore off after several months of therapy.

Secondly, many of the scientific trials involving fish oil used large (so-called pharmacological) doses of fish oil. Does fish oil still retain its beneficial effect in the relatively small doses that we recommend for the general population?

Finally, all of the evidence for fish oil so far has shown either that it lowers blood fats or that it reduces the risk of clotting in arteries. We have discussed a proven role in angina, but the conclusions from trials on patients where experts have looked at reduction in the risk of a heart attack are not so clear-cut. Although studies such as those by Nelson and Kromhout showed a reduced risk of heart attack in fish eaters, what they assessed was whether or not people who already ate fish ran less risk of a heart attack than did people who did not eat fish. This is not the same as changing the diet of a non-fish eater to that of a fish eater and assessing if the risk of a heart attack is reduced. The third question, and one which lies at the heart of this book, can be put like this. Can we show that by eating more oily fish, or by adding fish oil as a supplement to our diet, we can reduce the risk of a heart attack?

These three questions can only be answered by carefully evaluated scientific trial and assessment. Such trials have only just been brought to a conclusion, and we report on their findings in Chapter 6.

6

The Heart Attack Revolution

Dr Reg Saynor's seven-year study of the effects fish oil on heart patients

Becoming interested in the properties of fish oil was a fateful decision for Dr Saynor: it altered the course of his academic career and involved him in more than a decade of intensive research. Eventually this resulted in a large-scale study into the effects of fish oil on patients with raised blood fats, on patients with bad family health histories, and finally on the prevention of heart attack itself.

It was during the 1970s that he first heard the remarkable story of Hugh Sinclair, and in 1979 he saw this pioneer being interviewed on television. Sinclair impressed him, not only because he had exposed himself to personal danger in journeying twice to one of the most inhospitable places in the world, but also because he had financed his expedition himself. If Sinclair could work under the extreme difficulties of a tiny laboratory mounted on a dog sled, Dr Saynor was sure that he himself could set up some research, based on those early findings, in the comfortable surroundings of his laboratory in Sheffield. He had to admit that his initial reaction to Sinclair's diet of seal meat, fish and water was mixed. The diet obviously had fascinating potential effects, but it would have to be taken in a carefully controlled way. He asked himself how he could possibly get patients to eat this type of food. Quite apart from the impossibility of obtaining seal meat in Sheffield, it was hardly what they would normally eat and there would certainly be an emotional reaction to the idea of seals being slaughtered. Dr Saynor realized he must find another way.

Back in 1977 he had attended the first conference devoted to HDL-cholesterol as a risk factor in heart attacks, and had left determined to perform some research into this very interesting aspect of blood fats. Like all good research workers, he made himself the first volunteer to have his blood fats measured, only to discover to his horror that both his triglycerides and cholesterol were raised. Fortunately for him, his HDL-cholesterol was quite good, but he felt he had to do something quickly to get his blood fats back to normal.

For the first week or two he reduced them dramatically by almost starving himself, but it was clear that he could not keep up this self-mortifying exercise for very long. He changed to eating polyunsaturated fats, at the same time cutting back on the total amount of fat of any kind in his diet. He was thankful that his blood fats did not return to the previous very high levels, although even then he was still not altogether happy.

Then Dr Saynor heard of Hugh Sinclair's work, and it struck him that perhaps fish oil alone might be a substitute for the mixed fish and seal flesh in Sinclair's Eskimo diet. He went off to the local chemist's shop and bought a large bottle of cod liver oil from which he took one dessertspoonful every day. Imagine his delight when he found that, after only seven days of taking the oil, his triglyceride was almost down to normal. His cholesterol had not moved very much, but then he did not really expect it to alter because changes in cholesterol are slow and any anticipated change would take weeks or even months. His beneficial HDL-cholesterol had increased and this was a wonderful bonus, particularly since he had taken the oil for only seven days. Now he had to find some volunteers.

Cod liver oil first became popular almost a century ago because the high vitamin D content prevented rickets in children. But in our more affluent society it no longer has much place.

It was with considerable difficulty that he persuaded some colleagues to try the effect of fish oil on their blood fats. When you consider that even today much of the medical world still regards fish oil as a totally harmless and therefore ineffective sop to the credulous, you can imagine the kind of reaction he experienced.

In the end his colleagues were very cooperative – probably just to humour me, he thought – and he performed a small pilot study of fish oil's effectiveness over the very short time of six weeks. He felt vindicated when he saw their astonishment on observing the improvement to their blood fat levels.

At this stage Dr Saynor was no longer working with ordinary cod liver oil but with a purer oil which did not contain vitamins D and A. This was MaxEPA, supplied by courtesy of Seven Seas Health Care Ltd of Hull, the largest manufacturers of fish oil in the United Kingdom. They were sufficiently encouraged by his results to supply MaxEPA for a much larger study now to be performed on patients.

The next step was to enlist the help and cooperation of a colleague, Dr David Verel, a consultant cardiologist at the Northern General Hospital. Understandably, he was a little doubtful at first that fish oil would prove beneficial to his patients, but he agreed to refer patients to Dr Saynor for this treatment. Since that time Dr Verel has been very helpful and was co-author of many of the studies that Dr Saynor published.

The main study of the effectiveness of fish oil began in April 1980 and continued until May 1987. Dr Saynor was faced with some difficult decisions at this time. Since the pilot study had shown fish oil to be dramatically beneficial to people with raised blood fats, and since he was dealing with patients who not only had high blood fats but were a very high-risk group (many either suffered from angina or had already had one heart attack), he did not feel he could morally divide the patients and give half of them a placebo. Some of his medical colleagues have criticized this decision, but he felt he could only work according to his own sense of ethics. During those seven years, therefore, he gave fish oil to the whole of this high-risk group of 365 patients.

Out of these patients 153 had already suffered at least one heart attack, 58 suffered from angina without having had a heart attack, 14 had diabetes and the majority had significantly raised blood fats. A small number had had a previous stroke and 22 had narrowing of the arteries to their legs. Fifty-six had no history of arterial trouble at all, but had been referred to Dr Saynor simply because they had a bad family history of coronary heart disease. Before volunteers joined the study, its method and purpose were explained to them and they were permitted to take part or withdraw as they wished.

After the first month of treatment the triglyceride in all the patients had started to fall rapidly towards the normal level. One of the tenets of the study was that people participating in it should not make any changes to their diets, so any influence on their triglyceride levels from this means could be discounted.

From the very start Dr Saynor monitored their blood chemistry and full blood counts on each visit they made, carefully checking for any potential side-effects of the relatively high dose of fish oil they were taking (these patients were taking three times the dose we recommend in this book for general use). He was pleased to note that no side-effects ever occurred throughout this very long period of observation, whether complained of by the patients or observed in the blood tests. Medical colleagues were surprised by this, but it must be remembered that the fish oil used in the study, MaxEPA, is a natural product from a dietary source, the flesh of oily fish, which has been an integral part of the human diet for thousands of years.

Do the beneficial effects of fish oil wear off?

At this stage we can answer the first of those key questions posed at the end of Chapter 5. It is so essential to the theme of this book that we shall discuss it in some detail.

Throughout the full seven years of the study the triglyceride levels in Dr Saynor's patients' blood stayed low while they continued to take MaxEPA. If they stopped, their triglyceride levels rose again to the abnormally high level observed before treatment began. Two published scientific papers, one by Dr Schectman and the other by Dr Singer, queried the duration of effectiveness of fish oil, but these researchers' studies involved only sixteen and twelve patients respectively over periods of six and two months. Dr Saynor's results were obtained from a much larger group of patients over a much longer time, and they completely disproved this view.

Another difficulty with Dr Schectman's study was that he used not pure fish oil but one which had been extensively manipulated and chemically processed in order to increase certain of the Omega-3 fatty acids. In a letter to the *Lancet* in September 1989 Dr R. D. Rice explained the chemical changes that take place in this particular fish oil concentrate. He stated that the basic construction of the fish oil fatty acids is altered, and therefore results obtained with this substance may well differ from those of studies that use the more natural fish oils such as MaxEPA. Other researchers have also published details of differences between natural and processed oils. This is why we advise you to buy only pure oil that has not been chemically altered.

One fact that is very certain from Dr Saynor's study is that pure fish oil remains effective against raised blood fats for as long as you are taking it. Dr Saynor's findings have been confirmed in Japan by Dr Hamazaki and colleagues, in Australia by Dr L. A. Simons and colleagues, and here in the United Kingdom by a multi-centre study organized by Dr Paul Miller and colleagues.

The effects of fish oil on cholesterol

As stated in Chapter 4, cholesterol is one of the established risk factors in coronary heart disease; it was interesting to observe that in Dr Saynor's study the blood cholesterol level in his patients fell slowly but consistently, so that by the end of the first four years it was down 11 per cent. A small proportion of people may experience a slight rise in blood cholesterol if they take fish oil in addition to a diet rich in saturated fat. However, if the person's diet is modified to reduce saturated fat, as we recommend, and if most of the fat in the diet is in the form of polyunsaturates and monounsaturates, the effect of fish oil is to reduce the cholesterol substantially. You might say that this would happen anyway if the saturated fats were reduced, and you would be perfectly right, but research performed worldwide has shown that fish oil, which itself contains a unique mixture of polyunsaturates, will reduce the cholesterol even more effectively than other polyunsaturated oils when the two are taken together as part of your daily diet.

In Dr Saynor's study, the HDL-cholesterol concentration in his patients rapidly increased in a highly significant way and this was maintained throughout the seven-year period. You may recall that there is a link between triglyceride and HDL-cholesterol, so that when triglyceride comes down HDL-cholesterol increases. Only recently one medical colleague expressed the opinion that fish oil only raised HDL-cholesterol in patients who had abnormally high triglyceride, as if the increase in HDL-cholesterol in patients taking fish oil was just a secondary phenomenon. But Dr Saynor can confirm that fish oil raised the HDL-cholesterol in his patients regardless of whether their triglyceride was raised or normal to start with; in fact it raised the HDL-cholesterol in most of the people who took it. It is interesting that many other of our medical colleagues have now started to take fish oil, because they are already convinced of its efficacy.

The effects of fish oil on fibrinogen

Fibrinogen, as we explained earlier, is the most important blood-clotting protein in our circulation. However, if too much of it is present, as in cigarette smokers, the blood clots more readily and this constitutes an increased risk factor for heart attacks. The fibrinogen levels of all Dr Saynor's patients in the study were measured by an independent laboratory after every hospital visit, with fascinating results. The level started to decrease soon after they had started to take fish oil, and this reduction continued until their levels were normal. In this way fish oil was shown quite clearly and unequivocally to remove yet another of the risk factors.

Readers should be reassured that the reduction in fibrinogen was only into the normal range, and there was no tendency for the blood not to clot when it should – for instance after an accidental cut and so on. In other words there was considerable benefit once again, and no danger whatsoever.

Can it be shown that by deliberately increasing the amount of fish eaten, or by adding fish oil to the diet, the risk of a heart attack is reduced?

Leaving Dr Saynor's story again for a moment, let's look at the most vital question of all from Chapter 5. The answer, quite categorically, is Yes. The evidence for this was already good, if not solidly convincing, as recently as 1988 – about the time that the four major review papers described in Chapter 5 were written. There is now evidence from three further studies that proves the case beyond any reasonable doubt. Of Dr Saynor's 365 patients you will remember that 153 had already suffered a heart attack before participating in his study. In Sheffield, between 1980 and 1987 about 7 per cent per year of all such patients suffered a second heart attack. In the group investigated by his study only a little more than 1 per cent per year had another heart attack during the seven-year period. This is an extraordinary level of decreased risk, and by far the most important reduction reported in any of the studies of fish oil in relation to heart attack.

What about patients who had never had a previous heart attack? Let's look at another high-risk group, the fifty-eight angina sufferers. Remember that the majority of these patients, like those who had had a heart attack to start with, also had the high risk of raised blood fats when they began the study. Of these, none suffered a heart attack during the whole seven years. No more did patients without angina but who had a bad family history (many of whom again had raised blood fats) suffer a heart attack during the study.

The results of this large investigation over many years – the first of its kind in the world that used only fish oil as a therapy – can only be interpreted as very promising. The detailed scientific analysis is awaiting publication in the medical press at the time of writing (early 1990). It will be published under Dr Saynor's name and that of his colleague, Tim Gillott, who works in the Cardiothoracic Laboratory at the Northern General Hospital, Sheffield. Let's now see whether other experts and medical centres can confirm these important results.

The Burr study

In the last week of September 1989 the UK media were excited by the publication of a very important study by Dr Michael Burr and his colleagues based in the Medical Research Council Epidemiology Unit, Cardiff, and West Wales Hospital, Carmarthen. Their study subjects were 2033 men under the age of seventy, admitted to twenty-one different hospitals with a heart attack. Each man agreeing to take part in the study had his blood cholesterol measured at home, was weighed and was then randomly allocated either to have, or not to have, information on one of three special diets.

1. Advice on fats, designed to reduce saturated fat intake, aiming for a reduction in total fat intake to 30 per cent of total calories eaten, with equal quantities of polyunsaturates and saturates;

2. Fish advice, directing patients to eat at least two portions a week (200–400 g/7–14 oz) of fatty fish (mack-

erel, herrings, kippers, pilchards, sardines, salmon or trout); those who could not eat fish were allowed to take three capsules of MaxEPA a day instead; and

3. Fibre advice, increasing the intake of cereal fibre to 18 g (just under ¾ oz) a day.

Two variations of each type of diet (in other words they took it or they did not) would be coupled with either of the two variations of the other two dietary interventions. To understand this properly, if you tear three pieces of paper of different colours into halves, marking each with a Yes and a No, and then randomly allocate the six pieces so that any possible grouping of three will have either the Yes or the No in each colour, you will come up with eight possible combinations, including one group which receives all pieces marked 'No' (no dietary advice at all). Readers will quickly realize how difficult it is to set up a food intervention trial in order to achieve scientific credibility. In fact the researchers initially had to exclude over a thousand possible subjects because they already had definite ideas of their own about what parts of the above three dietary plan they wanted to follow.

Interestingly, when the results were looked at, those who had reduced their intake of fat showed no fall in the rate of further heart attacks – no more so than those who took extra fibre. The trial organizers thought this might be due to the fact that the blood cholesterol only fell by 3–4 per cent in these groups during the two years of the study. (Remember that they were allowed 50 per cent of dietary fat as saturates where we, for instance, recommend less than 40 per cent.) Dr Burr's conclusions were that only one group showed a major and significant fall in death rate from heart attack – those who ate a small amount of fatty fish per week or who took fish oil capsules. These patients had one-third fewer fatal heart attacks than any other group which did not eat fish.

Why the big difference in protection between Dr Saynor's and Dr Burr's studies?

This is uncertain, and will need confirmation from further research, but we suspect that it may be related to the dose of fish oil taken. The one-third lowering of the death rate in fish eaters is very similar to the protection rate from moderate fish eating in the Kromhout study described in Chapter 5. In both these studies the quantity of fish or fish oil taken was small. For instance, in Burr's study the effective dose of oil was about 3 g, the exact equivalent of the number of MaxEPA capsules given as a fish alternative, whereas in Dr Saynor's study the dose was 20 g to start with, followed by a maintenance dose of 10 g of oil. It is also instructive that this was the size of dose he had found to be the most effective in previous reported scientific studies.

The fact that fish or fish oil definitely does protect against heart attack, and the possibility that a gradual increase in protection can be achieved by increasing the dose, may have been confirmed by two more very large studies, one in Sweden and the other in the United States.

The Norell study

This was performed by Dr Stefan E. Norell, Professor Anders Ahlbom and colleagues of the Department of Epidemiology, National Institute of Enviromental Medicine, Stockholm. It looked at the possible link between fish consumption and mortality from coronary heart disease, and was reported in the *British Medical Journal* on 16 August 1986.

Over fourteen years they followed up 10,966 subjects; interestingly, these subjects were identical twins born in Sweden between 1886 and 1925. Each subject's average fish consumption in 1967 was categorized as high, moderate, low or none at all. Subjects who were already suffering from angina or coronary heary disease at the start of the study were excluded. The researchers looked at people who had died between 1969 and 1982 and related deaths from coronary heart disease to their consumption of fish.

The results showed not only a significant reduction in the risk of death from heart attack among the fish eaters, but also that there was a definite gradual lessening of risk as the consumption of fish rose. In other words, the results tended to confirm a relationship between the amount of fish eaten (or dose of fish oil) and the degree of protection from a fatal heart attack.

The American MRFIT study

Further confirmation of both the benefit of eating fish in this connection and of the suggestion that the benefit increases as the amount of fish eaten rises has now been provided by the MRFIT (pronounced Mr Fit) study in the United States.

The MRFIT is generally regarded as one of the most detailed and informative studies on heart attack ever performed. Its aim was not just to measure risk factors in heart attack but to intervene by reducing these risk factors and to see if this would prevent deaths. A very ambitious study, it was based in twenty-two clinical centres in the United States, where researchers screened men aged between thirty-five and fifty-seven and gathered together all those regarded as being at high risk of a heart attack, based on smoking, high blood pressure and high blood cholesterol. Over six to eight years 361,662 men were screened, from which 12,866 were selected for further study on the basis that they were thought to be at particularly high risk of heart attack. Approximately half were split at random into two study groups. One group received specific intervention to reduce smoking, blood pressure and blood cholesterol, while the second group were referred to their own doctors and returned to the study doctors annually for examination.

The results of fish consumption in this large trial have not yet been published but Dr Therese A. Dolecek, Assistant Professor in Public Health Sciences, Bowman Gray School of Medicine, North Carolina, presented their findings to the Second International Congress on Preventive Cardiology in June 1989. We are most grateful to Dr Dolecek for kindly giving us permission to refer to her presentation and allowing us access to her figures and findings. She performed a detailed analysis of the patients taking part in this study to see if fish eating produced an independent effect on death rate from heart attacks. She also analysed the oil content of the fish eaten and expressed her results in terms of the Omega-3 (n-3) polyunsaturated acids that were eaten in the form of fish.

First, and of considerable significance, the majority of American men seemed to eat very little oily fish. Two-thirds of the men participating in the trial were reported to eat an average of 0.1 g or less per day of Omega-3 fatty acid. When one considers that a single ounce of mackerel contains 0.6 g it is clear that Americans, like us in the UK, do not eat much oily fish.

Secondly, she reported 'a significant inverse relationship between Omega-3 fatty acid intake and CHD [coronary heart disease] mortality' – in other words, men who ate a small amount of fish had a significantly lower death rate from heart attacks. But she added another factor that tends to confirm the suggestion we made earlier in this chapter. 'There was a significant trend for a gradual decline in CHD mortality as fish protein intake increased.' In other words, another major study has suggested that the degree of protection increases with the quantity of fish oil consumed.

In case cynics should suggest that we have left out any important studies to suit our own argument, we can truthfully state that these are the only studies we could find in the world medical literature. It is not the purpose of this book to hype our subject or to persuade you with rhetoric. Our purpose is to give you proven scientific fact of the very highest credentials, and allow you to form your own opinion.

Case histories from Dr Saynor's experience

One lady had suffered from angina for a number of years. One of her favourite pastimes was walking in the Lake District, but now she was unable to enjoy this activity. Distressed by the fact that she was found not suitable for conventional treatment of her angina, she was referred to Dr Saynor. She started to take a dessert-spoonful of MaxEPA daily and within a few months was able to walk in the Lake District once more. Although she was still not able to tackle the steeper climbs, she coped very well with gentler slopes. Coronary heart disease is not just about the more dramatic aspect of life-and-death heart attacks.

The second case was a man of fifty who had very high blood fats and had already suffered one heart attack. His four brothers had all died from heart attacks before the age of fifty-two and he was understandably very worried. Once he began to take MaxEPA, his blood fats fell back to normal very quickly. That was in 1983. In 1989 he was still fit and active and claims to feel much better, from the point of view not only of his heart but of his general health as well.

7

What exactly is fish oil?

Fish oil, in its pure form, is the oil which is squeezed from the flesh (or muscle) of oily fish. It is different from cod liver oil which, as its name suggests, is squeezed from the liver and not the flesh. Cod liver oil is rich in vitamins D and A but less rich than pure fish oil in the essential fatty acids EPA and DHA.

We call it 'pure' fish oil to differentiate it from other processed fish oils which have undergone chemical and physical procedures to concentrate the oil and achieve higher levels of EPA and DHA. As we stated in Chapter 6, sometimes this processing can make important changes to the oil, so what we advise for our readers is very specifically pure fish oil. More details of what to buy, and the exact recommended dose, are given in Chapter 8, which also brings together all the dietary advice.

It is important to understand that all the medical trials we have discussed have involved either fish in the diet or fish oil. None of these trials has involved pure chemical preparations of EPA or DHA. It seems inevitable that future research will assess the effectiveness of these fatty acids as pure drugs, but it is premature to anticipate the results of such research. What we are saying is that, although we strongly suspect that EPA and DHA are the main active ingredients in fish oil, there are other ingredients in fish oil that could explain the beneficial effects on heart attack.

Dr Saynor's study, like many other important studies reported in the world medical literature, used MaxEPA, which, as stated earlier, has not been over-processed and does not contain chemically altered fatty acids as some other products do. The manufacturers have given us the following information on the approximate fatty acid content of their fish oil preparations.

Seven Seas liquid cod liver oil

EPA 9 per cent minimum, DHA 8 per cent minimum – this is equivalent to 393 mg EPA and 350 mg DHA in a 5 ml (or 4.6 g) teaspoonful. Note that not all teaspoons will hold 5 ml – this is a largish teaspoon size of the kind you get from the chemist with liquid medicines. If you are uncertain about the capacity of your spoons at home ask your chemist for a standard medicine spoon.

Seven Seas pure cod liver oil capsules

These have the same oil content as does the liquid cod liver oil, but note that the capsules only contain 0.3 g of oil each. You would have to take fifteen capsules to equal a single teaspoon of oil.

Seven Seas Pulse pure fish oil capsules

Each capsule contains 0.5 g of oil, which is richer in Omega-3 fatty acids than cod liver oil. Two capsules (or 1 g) contain 133 mg EPA and 86 mg DHA. It is best to take them in the morning before breakfast.

Seven Seas Pulse liquid emulsion

It is anticipated that an attractively flavoured liquid preparation of Pulse will soon be available, which would be an ideal way to take fish oil and would have some advantages over cod liver oil. This product will be approximately 50 per cent fish oil in emulsion with water and the concentration of EPA and DHA (added together to get total Omega-3 fatty acids) will be approximately halved in comparison with that of pure fish oil as in Pulse capsules. (See our recommended dose in Chapter 8.)

MaxEPA

This is available only on prescription for the medical condition known as hyper-triglyceridaemia. It comes in 1 g capsules, each of which contain 171 mg EPA and 114 mg DHA.

Other manufacturers' brands of fish oil or fish oil capsules

We have examined Seven Seas products first because they have been the main suppliers of oil for research in the United Kingdom and many other countries, and they have very high standards of purity, always rejecting fish from polluted waters. This does not mean that we view other manufacturers' brands as defective or unsuitable. But you really must take care when selecting a brand to buy. Choose from a well-established fish-oil food or drug manufacturer. If the label specifies the Omega-3 content in terms of ounces or grams of oily fish, refer to the tables on oily fish in Chapter 8. For example:

30 g/1 oz fresh salmon (but see the proviso on farm-harvested fish in Chapter 8) = approximately 0.4 g or 400 mg of Omega-3 fatty acids.

30 g/1 oz fresh mackerel = approximately 0.63 g or 630 mg of Omega-3 fatty acids.

30 g/1 oz fresh trout (but see the proviso on farm-harvested fish in Chapter 8) = approximately 0.17 g or

170 mg of Omega-3 fatty acids.

We recommend a dose of fish oil that will give you approximately 800 mg of Omega-3 fatty acids per day. Work out this figure by adding the EPA and DHA content of the oil you buy or from the fish you eat. Do not take more than 1000 mg (1 g) of Omega-3 fatty acids daily unless medically prescribed. Insist on pure fish oil – for example, a 5 ml teaspoonful of Pulse pure fish oil or a dessertspoon of Pulse emulsion daily. With other brands of pure fish oil, work out the correct dose from the manufacturer's statement of Omega-3 fatty acid content.

Safety first

In the doses we recommend we are not aware of any side-effect of fish oil. Nor would you anticipate any, since pure oil is exactly the same as the oil you eat in oily fish – though we would not, of course, recommend fish oil to somebody who was allergic to fish. In these small doses it seems unlikely you would experience an interaction with other medications such as aspirin or anticoagulant drugs. If this were so, then oily fish would have to be prohibited from the diets of such patients, which in practice is not the case.

Five million people take cod liver oil in the United Kingdom every year in very similar doses to those we recommend, without untoward effects. Since pure fish oil, as opposed to cod liver oil, first became available, this too has been taken by millions worldwide in this small dosage, and once again no serious problem has ever been reported. Fish oil in high dosage is a different matter, and we do not recommend high doses without medical supervision.

Many hundreds of medical studies have been performed on this aspect of the subject all over the world, and there have been few reports of any problems. In Dr Saynor's trial of 365 patients on moderately high doses over seven years there were no serious side-effects. In Dr Jorn Dyerberg's publications it is estimated that Eskimos consume some 14–15 g of Omega-3 fatty acids every day – a huge dose – and appear not only to be well on it but to be protected from several of the common serious diseases from which we in the Western world suffer. There are, however, some problems with high doses which, although not usually life-threatening, would have to be taken into consideration by doctors prescribing such doses.

Doses of fish oil as high as 20 g a day (and even higher relative doses of the Omega-3 concentrates) have been tested, and of course in these amounts factors such as calorie content have to be considered. Fish oil is a fatty substance, and therefore 1 g will add about 9 calories to our dietary total. A 5 ml teaspoon (less than 45 calories), or even a dessertspoon (less than 90 calories), does not amount to too many calories, but at 20 g and above calories would need to be taken into account.

One or two studies have found that diabetics may suffer slightly higher levels of blood sugar after taking large doses of fish oil – while other studies have shown dramatic improvements in diabetics taking the same doses. In the small doses we recommend, diabetics should experience no problems – and indeed it would be tragic if this simple therapy was denied to diabetic patients, who already suffer an increased risk of coronary heart disease. A study reported in 1989 by Schmidt and colleagues from Denmark, in the *Journal of Internal Medicine*, found that diabetics taking 4 g of fish oil a day, a very similar dose to that which we recommend for regular use, experienced significantly raised HDL-cholesterol, lowered triglyceride and an improved ratio of total cholesterol to HDL-cholesterol; and there were additional beneficial effects on their white blood cells.

Another problem that might arise with large doses of fish oil is in patients taking aspirin or blood-thinning treatment such as anticoagulant drugs. Although there have been few if any negative reports, a theoretical risk does exist in these cases. In Dr Saynor's trial, a number of patients did take aspirin or anticoagulants in addition to 10 g of MaxEPA daily, but none suffered any untoward effect such as excessive bruising or a tendency to bleed. Nevertheless caution is advisable, and we recommend that patients taking anticoagulant drugs such as warfarin should not take fish oil as a dietary supplement. The situation with regard to aspirin is uncertain and should be the subject of further medical study. Perhaps the wisest course would be for patients taking aspirin to take a small regular dietary intake of oily fish. An ounce of mackerel a day would be just right.

In practice, even reviewing the world literature, it is very difficult indeed to find any evidence against fish oil. There have been perhaps a thousand scientific investigations into its properties, yet only a handful have sounded any cautionary note. Even amongst these few, the query usually concerns the full beneficial effect.

Schacky, in the important review paper quoted above, concluded that the only side-effect observed in any study was a slight reduction in platelet count in the blood of two people taking huge overdoses (40 per cent of their total daily calories as fish oil). This effect completely disappeared when they reduced the amount of oil they were taking. Yetiv concludes, when considering the intake of preventive doses of fish oil in normal populations, that 'It is unlikely that such a low dose of n-3 fatty acid would have any significant deleterious effect.' Leaf and Weber say that if proper scientific studies were to show a benefit to the population from taking n-3 fatty acids, 'it would represent the most benign intervention in our pharmacopeia'. Taking the dose of pure fish oil as recommended in *The Eskimo Diet* is as safe as eating a small regular meal of oily fish.

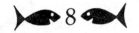

8

The Eskimo Diet

'In the immediate post-war period when meat supplies were scarce the consumption of fish increased sharply, but since then there has been a continuous decline, exacerbated recently by "cod wars", herring scarcities and vastly increased prices,' wrote Professor John Burnett in *Plenty and Want*. Fish is indeed a traditional part of Man's diet, but in many countries in the West we seem to have lost the habit.

During the evolutionary process our ancestors came from the sea, and the human foetus goes through a 'fishy' stage in which it has a tail and gills. Early human settlements tended to be about the coast or by lakes and rivers, and the living quarters of Stone Age Man tend to be recognizable from rubbish heaps full of shells. Dr Magnus Pyke, in his book *Man and Food*, remarks: 'Far inland, the bones of sea fish were discovered in the refuse heaps of the Old Stone Age cave dwellers in the Dordogne, dating from about 40,000 BC.'

In Elizabethan England half the total imports were fish, and much of the war at sea was fought over the cod-rich waters of Newfoundland. In Victorian times masters were warned against giving their apprentices salmon every day. Our rivers teemed with fish, and it was one of the cheapest sources of good nourishment. Is it mere accident that the nineteenth-century doctors hardly knew the meaning of the disease we now call a heart attack? They are admired today for their scrupulous accuracy in recording precise clinical descriptions of diseases, including some very rare conditions. Yet to them the very description of a heart attack as given earlier in this book – something you could hardly miss in a patient – was virtually unknown. Then came the twentieth century.

In *Diet of Man: Needs and Wants*, Lord Trenchard gives a table of fish consumption in the United Kingdom this century. Between 1909 and 1913 an average member of the population, including the elderly and children, ate 41 lb of fish a year. You hardly need your pocket calculator to work out that if this were fatty fish, it would be twice the dietary intake recommended in this book. From 1913 to 1941 the consumption dwindled to a third as much, and then rose sharply towards the end of the war, only to continue the previous long decline from 1950 onwards. That the situation in the United States is similar can be seen from the basic data of the MRFIT study reported in Chapter 6. Once again, during and immediately after the Second World War the death rate from heart attack remarkably and inexplicably dipped. The same thing happened in Norway, where during the war there was a similar rise in fish consumption.

Our approach in this book has been explanation rather than persuasion. In the end, given the facts, only you can decide what to do for yourself and your family. That is why we have devoted almost half the book to explanation of what a heart attack is and how it might be best dealt with, and to the scientific exploration of the wonderful possibilities of fish and fish oil. Now we ask you to arrive at your own considered conclusion – do you believe in the Eskimo Diet or not?

Our strategy aims at moderation in both diet and lifestyle. Although fat is perceived as the enemy, we need a reasonable amount of it in our diets to avoid a deficiency of the fat-soluble vitamins A and D. We would

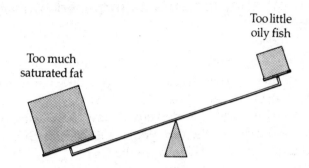

Too little
oily fish

Too much
saturated fat

Figure 10   *Getting the balance wrong*

therefore suggest a common-sense approach, based on a re-establishment of what we call the strategic balance. A vital factor was missing from our diet, the right-hand side of the balance, as illustrated (see *Figure 10*). In our opinion, the balance of the average Western diet has become seriously upset. It should not prove very difficult – and we hope it might even prove pleasurable – to redress this (see *Figure 11*).

Plan of the Eskimo Diet

1. Eat oily fish at least twice a week, and supplement this with fish oil on the days you do not eat fish.

2. Keep the amount of saturated fat in your diet low, replacing it with polyunsaturates and monounsaturates.

3. Eat more fibre, and less sugar and salt.

4. Enjoy a drink, but not too often.

5. Above all, make your diet varied and enjoyable – increase, rather than decrease, the happiness factor in your life.

Fish oil supplements as opposed to eating fish

We would recommend that your diet includes as much natural food as possible, and that you take your fish oil in the form of eating oily fish. This is not only very palatable but has the added advantage of replacing meat as a main dish on the day you eat it, so reducing your intake of saturated fat into the bargain.

However, we recognize that many people do not like eating fish. Taste is a very difficult thing to change, and many of those responsible for shopping and preparing meals will find that they can only introduce more fish in a gradual way, re-educating the palates of their families. For somebody who cannot or does not wish to eat oily fish, fish oil is the only way to take the essential Omega-3 fatty acids.

Dosages for different people

1. If you eat a small quantity of oily fish daily, say a minimum of 30 g/1 oz mackerel or the equivalent in any other fish, you do not need supplements.

Figure 11   *Getting the balance right*

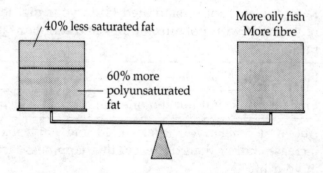

40% less saturated fat

60% more polyunsaturated fat

More oily fish
More fibre

2. For people who eat oily fish at least twice a week, we would recommend a 5 ml teaspoonful of pure fish oil daily or a dessertspoon of 50 per cent oil and water emulsion on the days you do not eat oily fish.

3. People who eat little or no oily fish need to take all their Omega-3 fatty acids as supplements. A teaspoonful of oil daily or a dessertspoonful of a 50 per cent emulsion would be sufficient to provide our recommended 800 mg a day.

Which are the oily fish?

Different types of fish contain very different amounts of the protective oils. For instance, cod, haddock and plaice, the favourites in the UK diet, are all poor providers of fish oil. Fish can no more manufacture the essential EPA and DHA fatty acids than we can. They obtain their supplies from plankton, the micoscopic organisms that float in the sea. Because of this, fish that have been bred in farms and fed soybean or other plant seeds or grains may be very poor suppliers of fish oil. As a general rule, fish netted from the sea or open rivers and lakes are the best providers.

Our means of cooking the fish also has an effect on the oily content. Frying removes some of the oils from the fish. Grilled, baked, poached or lightly boiled fish offer the best guarantee of goodness. Prolonged boiling removes the oils from the flesh, and this can be a problem with some brands of tinned tuna. If you like this fish, it may be best to buy it canned in brine.

The following table, modified from an authoritative report entitled 'Provisional tables on the content of Omega-3 fatty acids and other fat components of selected sea-foods' by Hepburn, Exler and Weihrauch, and published in the *Journal of the American Dietetic*

Association, lists the beneficial oils in most common fish and some varities. The fish are grouped in three sections: highly beneficial, moderately beneficial and poorly beneficial. Within the sections we have listed them according to the fatty acid content per 100 g/3½ oz.

Many readers will be experienced in buying and cocking fish. If not, we suggest you develop your skills with the more common highly beneficial varieties; then you can start to experiment, and ask your fishmonger about some of the less common types of fish.

The tables all assume fresh fish and uncooked weight.

Fish with a high fatty acid content (most beneficial)

Type of fish	Approximate n-3 fatty acid content as grams contained in 100 g/3½ oz of fish
Mackerel	2.2
Spiny dogfish	2.0
Herrings and sardines	1.7
Pilchards	1.7
Tuna (bluefin)	1.6
Trout (lake)	1.6
Sturgeon (Atlantic)	1.5
Salmon	1.4
Anchovies	1.4
Sprats	1.3
Bluefish	1.2
Mullet (unspecified)	1.1
Halibut	0.9
Bass (striped)	0.8
Trout (rainbow)	0.6
Trout (Arctic char)	0.6
Trout (brook)	0.6
Mullet (striped)	0.6
Oysters	0.6
Carp	0.6

Type of fish	Approximate n-3 fatty acid content as grams contained in 100 g/3½ oz of fish
Squid (short-finned)	0.6
Tuna (skipjack)	0.5
Tuna (unspecified)	0.5
Sturgeon (common)	0.4
Squid (Atlantic)	0.4
Bass (freshwater)	0.3
Squid (unspecified)	0.3

Fish with a medium fatty acid content (moderately beneficial)

Type of fish	Approximate n-3 fatty acid content as grams contained in 100 g/3½ oz of fish
Hake (unspecified)	0.5
Mussels (blue)	0.5
Periwinkles	0.5
Shark	0.5
Catfish (brown bullhead)	0.5
Pollock	0.5
Hake (Pacific)	0.4
Sea bass	0.4
Shrimps	0.4
Crab	0.4
Perch (white)	0.4
Catfish (channel)	0.3
Perch (yellow)	0.3
Perch (ocean)	0.2
Hake (Atlantic)	0.1

Fish with a poor fatty acid content (least beneficial)

Type of fish	Approximate n-3 fatty acid content as grams contained in 100 g/3½ oz of fish
Pike (wall-eye)	0.3
Clams	0.3
Cod (Atlantic)	0.3
Cod (Pacific)	0.2
Plaice (European)	0.2
Scallops	0.2
Flounder	0.2
Lobster	0.2
Eel	0.2
Pike (northern)	0.1
Abalone	0.1
Haddock	0.1

From this comprehensive list it should be possible to devise many colourful and appetizing main meals. Try in time to extend your range of dishes and tastes, and remember that what seems strange and new may need several attempts with different recipes before you really make the best of its attractiveness and flavour. All the recipes in Chapter 9 have been devised by our wives and tested by us – they are delicious, and we hope you enjoy them too.

We would recommend that you aim for fish in the first two categories, in other words those with high and medium fatty acid content. This does not mean that you should stop enjoying the popular white fish in the low fatty acid category, such as cod, haddock and plaice. These fish would all have a role on those days when the aim is to reduce your intake of saturated fat.

A word about cooking fish and accompanying sauces

Avoid cooking fish in butter or other animal fats. Frying removes the very oils we need, so grill, bake, poach or lightly boil the fish, or else eat it cold as with smoked salmon and mackerel.

Sauces undoubtedly give colour and additional flavour to fish, but in Britain we tend to make them with saturated fats such as butter and cream. In countries such as Portugal, however, where fish has remained the national dish, the traditional mouth-watering sauces are often quite different from ours and vegetable-based. They are brightly coloured (instead of the bland white sauce on white fish we favour) and have been cooked in unsaturated vegetable oil. Make a point of including olive oil in your meals whenever possible.

Vegetable sauces are made essentially from tomatoes (fresh or tinned), onions, herbs, olive oil, mushrooms, peppers and, if you like it, garlic. It is quite easy to think up other ideas for ingredients yourself. The key is a very juicy mix, cooked in vegetable oil. Low-fat sauces, incidentally, tend to be cheaper than high-fat ones. Why not experiment with the sauces yourself – try more than one with a meal at first, and discover which is most to the family's taste.

Cutting down on saturated fat

Saturated fat usually arrives in the shopping basket in the form of animal and dairy produce, but it also has many more subtle forms. Cholesterol tends to come with saturated fat, but certain foods such as eggs, liver, kidneys and fish roe are very high in cholesterol while not so high in saturated fat. The following list contains some unexpected exceptions in categories which are otherwise good for you. Watch out for them. Everyone will find some items on the list which they are fond of: remember that you are not 'forbidden' to eat these, but you should try to reduce them to a minimum and allow yourself an occasional treat.

Foods containing saturated fat

Meat and meat products, such as beef, lamb, pork, suet, lard and dripping, are some of the chief sources. Very high saturated fats are found in brisket, corned beef, spare ribs, bacon, sausages and luncheon meats, and in fast foods such as hot dogs and hamburgers. High-cholesterol foods otherwise include liver, fish roes and – you might be amused to hear – caviar.

Dairy products, another major source of saturated fat, include full-cream and half-cream milk (but not skimmed), soft cheeses, butter, certain yogurts (not the low-fat varieties), certain ice creams (though you can get reduced-fat ice creams), custard made with full-cream milk, condensed milk, dried and evaporated milk. Also high in saturated fat are cheese spreads and dips.

Although the meats of chicken and turkey are excellent for being low in saturated fat, certain poultry, mainly duck and goose, are high in saturated fat. There is saturated fat in the skin of all poultry, including chicken and turkey.

Some vegetable oils, in particular coconut and palm oil, are surprisingly high in saturated fat (see page 117) and should therefore be reduced considerably or avoided altogether.

Less obvious sources of saturated fat include cakes, doughnuts, pancakes, waffles, biscuits, chocolates (cocoa butter), cooking fats, hard margarines, sauces and puddings. Sauces in particular must be watched, as explained above. Wherever possible, substitute natural yogurt or skimmed milk for cream, and the right kinds of vegetable oil, polyunsaturated margarine or low-fat spread for butter.

Remember that you can lose some of the benefit gained by a reduced intake of saturated fat if you use high-fat sauces or nibble high-fat snacks at lunchtime, or, most seductive of all, in that final snack before bedtime. A bonus from cutting down on saturated fat snacks is weight reduction, since fat contains more calories than any other food source. Because of the dangers of these regular snacks, it is well worth while setting your mind to alternative low-fat snacks and – more importantly still – making sure they are easily available for hungry mouths at the most dangerous times of day. Another great temptation, which we all suffer from, is rushing to find a quick bite and ruining a whole day's careful eating with a moment's temptation.

As a general rule of thumb, oils, fats, margarines and foods of vegetable origin will be rich in polyunsaturates and will usually contain no saturated fat. This is the basis of vegetarian diets, but vegetarian does not necessarily mean healthy, since diary produce in particular, which tends to be a main ingredient of many vegetarian diets, contains very high proportions of saturated fats.

Another general rule is that cholesterol in our diet is usually bound up with saturated fat so that a diet low in saturated fat is also a low-cholesterol diet. There are a few exceptions to this – eggs, for instance, contain a lot of cholesterol in the yolk. Another food whose cholesterol content worried people for a time is shellfish – but in fact their initial concern may have been exaggerated. While this may still be controversial, the actual weight of shellfish per individual portion is usually small, so that there is no real worry about cholesterol content unless somebody is on a very strict low-cholesterol diet. This type of diet does not apply generally and would only be prescribed to those rare individuals with very high blood cholesterols which are resistant to changes in diet.

Monounsaturates

Oleic acid is the main example, and it derives its name from the oil in which it is commonly found, olive oil. Olive oil (and whole olives) is the best source, but others include avocados, peanuts, certain nut and seed oils and, perhaps surprisingly, meat fat, butter and eggs. On the continent, particularly in France and other Mediterranean countries where heart attacks are much less common than in the UK, it is the custom both to cook in olive oil and to place olive oil on the table for liberal consumption. While using olive oil in cooking is purely a question of practice and thinking about it in advance, its use in salads, for instance, is a question of taste. It would be a very good thing to encourage this taste. There is gathering evidence that olive oil does reduce the risk of a heart attack, and we might as well give it the benefit of the doubt.

Polyunsaturates

Polyunsaturates generally have a cholesterol-lowering effect and this is one reason why they are preferred to saturates. An additional very important reason is that, while they are fats and therefore contain important nutritional substances such as the fat-soluble vitamins, they are not thought to have any risk in connection with heart attacks. Therefore they are seen as an ideal replacement for the saturated fat that needs to be reduced in the Eskimo Diet. Fat should give you only about 30 per cent of your total calories, and of this less than 40 per cent should come from saturates.

It may help you to understand those figures in the nutritional information on food labels if we say that this means you take about 50 g/1¾ oz of polyunsaturates and monounsaturates combined per day and a maximum of 30 g/1 oz of saturates. Of course people don't go about all day calculating exact grams of fats, but a little time spent thinking about it or looking at labels in the super-market will give you a surprising amount of information.

The EPA and DHA fatty acids in fish oil (collectively known as the Omega-3 or n-3 content) are examples of very special polyunsaturates. But those found in abund-ance in fresh vegetables (known as Omega-6 and non-fish oil type Omega-3 fatty acids) have special benefits of their own. These polyunsaturates are found in some vegetable oils, such as sunflower, soya, corn and grape-seed oil, in soft margarines made from these oils (look on the packaging and it will say 'high in polyunsaturates') and in nuts. The following table illustrates the main oils and fats and their average saturate contents. Nearly all of the rest of the oil or fat is in the form of monounsaturates and polyunsaturates. From a quick glance down this table you can check the cooking oil you use and choose a better one if necessary.

Oils

	Grams of saturates per 100g/3½ oz
Coconut oil	85
Palm oil	49
Peanut/groundnut oil	19
Wheatgerm oil	19
Safflower oil	16
Soya oil	14
Sesame seed oil	14
Grapeseed oil	14
Blended cooking oil (poor quality)	14
Olive oil	13.4
Sunflower oil	13
Corn oil	11
Walnut oil	9
Blended cooking oil (good quality)	7

The next table shows you the fat breakdown of solid cooking fats. Notice that all of these contain more saturates than the vegetable oils commonly used in cooking, but once again there are huge variations between, say, solid sunflower oil fat and beef dripping. Once again, nearly all the remaining weight of the cooking fat is monounsaturate and polyunsaturate.

Solid Cooking Fats

	Grams of saturates per 100 g/3½ oz
Dripping (solid beef fat)	59
Solid white cooking fat	47
Lard (pork fat)	38
Solid vegetable fat	26–50
Sunflower oil solid cooking fat	20

What about eggs?

Eggs are an excellent source of many nutrients. Unfortunately the yolk is high in cholesterol and because of this we advise you to limit your consumption to about three a week. One or two of these will probably come in the form of cooked food, but the remainder can be enjoyed as a boiled or poached egg (not fried) for breakfast.

Margarine versus butter

Should we eat butter or margarine? What about these newer butters which claim to be high in polyunsaturates? If you are the shopper in your family, how do you interpret the labels on these kinds of food so you know what you are giving your family to eat? Remember that, as always, it is a question of quantity of saturated fat eaten rather than percentages. If you really like butter, full-cream milk, cheese, chocolate and so on, you can indulge yourself a little – but do it with knowledge of what you are doing and restrict the saturated fat to an average of less than 30 g/1 oz a day (see Chapter 7). If you eat more one day, take less the next – so over, say, a week you keep it under control.

It is of course much easier to control quantity when the percentage of saturated fat is low, and this is the reason why polyunsaturated margarines have become so popular. We have examined the information provided on butter and margarine packets, and these are examples of what we have found.

Interpreting the nutritional information on butter and margarine

The butters and margarines we looked at were picked at random from our local supermarket, and we do not recommend these any more than other brands. What we do advise is that you insist that the food you buy does carry this kind of nutritional labelling, particularly when there is substantial fat present. Only by you, the customer, insisting will manufacturers and retailers get the message that you have an absolute right to know what you are eating.

Ordinary butter
Reading the label on ordinary butters tells you little, because they don't usually say what quantity or percentage of saturates they contain. On average the saturated composition of butter is about 60 per cent. The label will probably just tell you if it is salted or not.

Low-fat butters and margarines

Golden Churn

Nutritional composition per 100 g/3½ oz

Energy (i.e. calories)	680 kcal (also expressed as 2830 kJ, i.e. kilo-Joules)
Protein	0.3 g
Carbohydrate (i.e. sugars, starches, etc.)	1.0g
Fat	75g
(of which saturates)	14 g
Salt	1.8 g

In other words, this brand of reduced-fat butter contains just 14 per cent of its weight as saturated fat in comparison with about 60 per cent in ordinary butter. We have to assume that the remainder of the fat content must be mainly polyunsaturates and possibly some monounsaturates. It would therefore be much easier to keep to less than 30 g/1 oz a day of saturated fat if you ate this product.

Flora

Nutritional composition per 100 g/3½ oz

Energy (calories)	740 kcal (3041 kJ)
Protein	0.3 g
Carbohydrate	1.4 g
Fat	80 g
(of which saturates)	14 g
Polyunsaturates	42 g

Notice first that the percentage of saturates in its total weight is the same as Golden Churn, at 14 per cent. But Flora, unlike Golden Churn, tells us the actual proportion as polyunsaturates, 42 per cent. The information on the pack does not, however, tell us what makes up the remainder of the fat (24 per cent of the total).

St Ivel Gold

Nutritional composition per 100 g/3½ oz

Energy (calories)	390 kcal
Protein	6.5 g
Carbohydrate	2.0 g
Fat	39 g
(of which saturates)	10.5 g
Salt	1.3 g

This brand has a much lower calorie content than the previous two and the saturated fat percentage is slightly lower. In fact all three of these low-fat brands are considerably lower than ordinary butter in saturated fat. Choosing between them, or any other brand, is a matter of taste and concern for the other contents, such as calories and salt.

All three brands also give useful information on where the fat contents come from. They mention vegetable oils such as sunflower oil, hydrogenated vegetable oils (these mean saturated fat), skimmed milk, whey, lecithin (a chemical related to fat), flavourings, natural colours and vitamins.

The following table will give you a very clear idea of the average fat contents of different margarines and butter. It is again expressed as grams per 100 g/3½ oz, but the figures are very close to percentages of total weight. This table also includes a breakdown of the unsaturates into monounsaturate and polyunsaturate to give you some idea of what really does go into the composition of margarines and butter. Your guide is still, of course, the column headed 'saturates'.

Margarine, butter and low-fat spreads

| | Grams per 100 g/3½ oz | | |
	Saturates	Mono-unsaturates	Poly-unsaturates
Butter	49–60	27	2
Hard table margarine	35	32	4
Hard cooking margarine	31	32	12
Soft table margarine	22	39	15
Soya margarine	17	32	27
Sunflower margarines	14	24	42
Low-fat spreads	8	17	13

It is clear that you could eat five or six times the amount of low-fat spread as butter and only add the same amount of saturated fat to your intake. This principle also applies to hidden fats in cooking, or in bought foods such as confectionery and cakes. Keep an eye on the ingredients, which should be clearly stated on the packaging. Low-fat spreads are not suitable for cooking, but polyunsaturated margarines, such as sunflower margarines, often are.

A simple idea of how much saturated fat you or your family are already eating can be assessed by looking through your usual week's shopping at the supermarket. You'll only need to do it once to get a good general idea. Add up the saturated fat on the packages and cans, add to this an estimate from the meat, poultry and fish you buy, and make sure to include milk, cheese and any fast foods or items such as sweets and chocolates that are bought casually. Remember our guideline for daily total fat is about 80 g/3 oz and for saturated fat about 30 g/1 oz.

The quality of margarines can vary a lot, depending

on what type of oil they are prepared from. Sometimes the use of the term 'vegetable oil' can be misleading. If the manufacturer uses the term 'hydrogenated vegetable oil' or 'hydrolyzed vegetable oil' this means that an unsaturated vegetable oil has been converted into saturated fat by hydrogenation. The cheaper margarines and hard cooking fats may contain palm oil and animal fats, and this explains their much higher saturated fat content.

The harder a margarine or cooking fat is at room temperature, the higher the content of saturated fat. Vegetable margarines often need to be kept in the fridge, but don't let them get too hard since a softer spread goes further and this too helps to reduce the actual quantity eaten. Remember also that if you don't always win the war on saturated fat, you will still gain considerable benefit by eating more fish and by taking fish oil.

What sort of milk should I buy?

Have a look at the following list of saturated fat contents in a single bottle of different types of milk.

Milk

	Grams of saturates per pint
Full-cream milk (gold top)	28
Ordinary dairy milk (silver top)	22
Semi-skimmed milk (red-striped top)	11
Skimmed milk (blue-hatched top)	1

The message is obvious. When you first change to skimmed milk, you miss the creamy taste and texture, but within a few weeks you will discover you prefer the taste of your breakfast cereal or tea unclogged by the overpowering richness of the cream content. Once again it is a question of quantity consumed over twenty-four hours; But taking skimmed milk allows you to drink as much as you like – and we are all for making life as easy as possible.

Condensed milk and evaporated milk contain a lot of fat, so avoid them whenever possible.

You will hear some people say that skimmed milk is nothing more than water or that it has had all of the goodness taken out of it. This is not true. Skimmed milk contains the same amount of calcium and milk protein as ordinary milk. But do not give skimmed milk to babies or very young children for whom milk is a major part of their daily diet. Under these circumstances the saturated fat is needed for a proper calorie intake and must not be left out.

But I love thick cream!

Most of us do. A tip for getting over the withdrawal symptoms is to use low-fat yogurt instead of cream whenever possible. Greek yogurt is particularly smooth and creamy textured. If you do use cream, use single rather than double. Beware of artificial creams, which often contain just as much saturated fat as real cream.

Another tip is the notion of 'little treats' – you can be allowed full cream just now and then. Remember it is always a question of overall intake, perhaps over a week rather than a day. If you've kept fairly well to the diet for a week you could be allowed a treat at Sunday lunchtime, or on a special evening out.

What about cheese?

Go for the ones with the least fat – see the general guide to fat intake in table below. The joy of an occasional treat need not be denied.

Cheeses are natural foods, eaten since prehistoric times. If you like a particular cheese, or cheese in general, there is no reason why you shouldn't continue to do so. It is merely a question of how much you eat and how often. You need to take two factors into consideration: fat content (both total and saturated) and salt content.

A portion of cheese eaten with biscuits at the end of a meal can vary from about 30 g/1 oz to more than about 125 g/4 oz. Under ordinary circumstances a small portion can easily be accommodated within the recommended daily total and saturated fat limits. 125 g/4 oz of a cheese such as Cheddar, on the other hand, will equal two-thirds of your daily recommended intake of saturated fat. If you like large portions of cheese, try to develop a taste for a low-fat kind or reduce the alternative sources of saturated fat in your diet, for example meat and other dairy produce.

When preparing sandwiches, you may find you can use less cheese if you buy ready-cut slices.

Here is a list of the total and saturated fat content of some common cheeses – but remember that these are for larger portions of cheese than most people eat. Note also that the difference between 'low-fat' and other kinds is huge, and that the 'medium-fat' category is much closer to 'high-fat' than to 'low-fat'.

Cheese	Total fat content (g) per 100 g/ 3½ oz	Saturated fat content (g) per 100 g/ 3½ oz
Low-fat		
Cottage		
creamed	4.8	2.8
1% fat	1	1
2% fat	2	1.5
Curd cheese	1	0
Edam, low-fat (11%)	11.3	6.5
Quark skimmed milk	0.3	less than 0.3
Shape cottage	0.5	less than 0.5
Medium-fat		
Cheese spread	21	14
Delight	17	10
Feta	21.4	14
Mild goat's cheese (medium-fat, soft cheese)	18.1	12.6
Mozzarella		
part skimmed	17.5	10.5
full fat	20	12.7
Shape low-fat	16.5	10
Tendale	15	10
High-fat		
Brie	28	17.5
Camembert	24.5	14
Cheddar	33	22
Cheshire	31.5	21
Cream cheese	47	25
Edam	28	17.5
Emmental	28	17.5
Gouda	28	17.5
Gruyère	31.5	17.5
Kraft slices (Cheddar)	24	16
Parmesan	28	17.5
Roquefort	30.5	17.5
Stilton	40	26

It is relatively easy to estimate your consumption of fat from raw cheese, but the task is less easy when it comes to cheese-based dishes in ready-cooked foods or in restaurants. These can be a major source of saturated fat. The following table assumes average restaurant portions and that the cheese is a high-fat variety.

Type of Food	Total fat content (g)	Saturated fat content (g)
Cheese sandwich	25	15
Cheeseburger		
regular	13	6.7
quarter-pounder burger with cheese	26.4	14
Cheesecake	21	12
Cheese fondu	18	9
Cheese sauce	17	9
Cheese straws	18	8

Another high saturated fat source is cheese dips, which are often made with sour cream, cream cheese, Cheddar cheese or blue cheese. It is far better to make dips with low-fat yogurt or low-fat cottage cheese. Low-fat yogurt in particular makes a lovely full-flavoured dip and you can add your own herbs and spices.

Let's talk about meat

Meat, like dairy produce, is one of the highest sources of saturated fat in our diet. In the Third World, which may approximate to the difficult circumstances of our ancestors, very little meat is eaten. This is because meat is relatively expensive and vegetables are much cheaper and more plentiful. If we compare our consumption of meat today to that in nineteenth-century Britain, when heart attacks were very uncommon, it is much higher. We also eat less fish and bread.

We are not suggesting that you eat no meat. On the contrary, we think that you could eat it about twice a week as a main meal, which leaves room for some meat in sandwiches and snacks perhaps another twice a week. Here in the UK butchers tend to cut meat across the muscle fibres (across the grain), which tends to keep the fat, which is trapped between muscle bundles. On the continent, paricularly in countries such as France, which has a lower incidence of coronary heart disease, butchers tend to cut meat so as to remove any fat between the fibres. When you buy meat pick the leanest cut you can find, and before cooking it cut off any fat. Do not add lard or dripping. Learn techniques for trimming off surplus fat from raw meat and scooping off liquid fat during cooking.

What's so special about chicken and turkey?

If you look at the meat in chicken, turkey or game, you will not find the thick white fat that you usually find between the muscle bundles and over the surface of red meat. Most of the fat in poultry is under the skin. There is a small amount in between the muscle of the meat, but this is very easily removed. Because of this, we encourage you to eat poultry say twice a week. But remember to remove the skin (and with it, therefore, most of the fat).

What's not so special about duck and goose?

Ironically, they are high in saturated fat and cholesterol, and so we need to treat them as high-fat meats.

Fat content of meat and fish

In general about 40–50 per cent of the fat in meat is saturated. In chicken this is about 25 per cent, which is much the same level as in fish. Yes, fish does contain saturates too – but the relatively low levels are more than balanced by the polyunsaturates.

Will I become deficient in iron if I cut down on meat?

This is a very good question, since meat and liver are good sources of iron in the diet. To reduce saturated fat we have suggested that you only eat red meat in a main meal twice a week, so the possibility of not eating enough iron is a real one, especially for women before the menopause.

Our body only takes in iron at a very low rate because in larger amounts it is toxic within the body. This means we need a good *steady* supply of iron in our diet. One way round this is to take a small dose of iron in the form of tablets such as Iron Jelloids. But be cautious. Many people don't tolerate iron tablets very well, and a normal healthy man or woman should only require a maximum of about 20 mg a day in his or her diet. In fact we absorb only a tiny proportion of this, perhaps 1–2 mg, but we need the excess to 'make' the body take in this small natural requirement. We would recommend that you to take your non-meat iron in the form of natural food rather than tablets – it is quite easy.

Iron is found in a wide variety of foods other than red meat or liver. Fish contains about a third of the iron level of red meat. Many vegetables contain good levels, for instance lentils by dry weight contain twice as much weight for weight as red meat, but it is not taken in quite as well by the body. Examples of excellent vegetable sources include lentils, kidney beans and pulses generally, baked beans, haricot beans and spinach. Make sure you include lots of these types of vegetable in your diet.

One excellent way of taking iron may well surprise you – fortified breakfast cereals. These have the additional advantage of containing other essential vitamins. Weetabix contains twice as much weight for weight as meat, All-bran about three times as much, Shredded Wheat about a third more and Bran Flakes almost seven times as much, all of these by dry weight of the cereal. Read your cereal packet and see how much iron it contains. It is quite possible that you can get all the iron you need in a day from your breakfast cereal alone.

More insidious foods that contain a lot of fat

These are often children's favourites – remember that here in the UK the first signs of atheroma in our arteries, the so-called fatty streaks, can be seen even in the arteries of our children. These hidden fats are to be found in crisps, chocolates, cakes, confectionery and biscuits.

Here again, we don't encourage fanaticism. The occasional little treat is what life is about – and you will find that crisps and cakes, for instance, are now available cooked with polyunsaturated oil, margarine or cooking fat. Try to reduce the amount you buy, and when you do buy go for those with a lower saturated fat content.

General tips on cutting down fat in cooking

Some of the ideas in this section were inspired by the excellent booklet *Guide to Healthy Eating,* published by the Health Education Authority. This is available free of charge from your local Health Education Unit, and we would like to thank the publishers for permission to borrow some of their ideas.

Often you can cut down saturated fat considerably simply by cooking differently. Take potatoes, for instance. If you eat them as a generous portion of chips you will consume approximately 240 calories containing 14 g of saturated fat (about half your daily allowance). With baked potato, you eat half the calories and virtually no saturated fat. But if you stuff the baked potato with sour cream and chives, you double the calories and ruin the whole plan by adding 24 g of saturated fat from the cream. On the other hand if you use low-fat cottage cheese to stuff your potato, you reduce the additional calories by more than half and you reduce the saturated fat to negligible amounts. Here are some useful tips in keeping saturated fat down while still enjoying your food.

Avoid frying whenever you can. Grill, bake, poach or boil whenever possible. Another tip when frying is that you should only fry food with a high water content, say chips for example, twice or three times in the same oil. The process of frying 'hydrolyses' the vegetable oil, converting the polyunsaturates to saturates.

Casseroling or stewing is an excellent alternative way to cook meat and it means you can buy cheaper cuts of meat – but remember always to *buy lean and remove as much fat as possible, even after cooking*. Place your cooked casserole in the fridge when cool. Once it has got quite cold the fat will have risen and solidified and you can break it off like ice on a pond. Then reheat your casserole when you want to eat it. Casseroles usually taste better when made in advance, anyway. After roasting, pour the meat juices from the roasting tin into a saucepan, add very cold water and put it into the fridge until the fat solidifies and floats on the surface. It is then relatively easy to spoon off the solid saturated fat and make your gravy from the rest. Another technique for separating off the fat is to add a trayful of ice cubes to the gravy, which serves the dual purpose of solidifying the fat and diluting the remains of fat in the gravy.

When *mashing potatoes*, avoid adding butter or margarine. You can add skimmed milk, which makes the potatoes very tasty and adds hardly any saturated fat at all.

When *preparing pâtés*, use skimmed milk or low-fat yogurt instead of butter, margarine or cream.

Chicken and poultry: casserole rather than roast, which allows you to take the skin off first. Remember that most of the saturated fat in chicken and poultry is just under the skin and comes away with it.

With *minced meat*, it is hard to tell how much fat there is in it. Even mince that looks quite red is usually quite fatty. Choose your own lean cut of meat and either mince it yourself or have it minced at the butcher's. There are several techniques for removing most of the fat. For example, just heat the mince in a pan, scoop it up with a draining spoon and put it on kitchen paper to drain off the fat. Then put the mince back into a clean pan and cook it in the normal way. Even simpler, heat up the mince in a pan and drain away the fat as it comes away from the meat.

Grill, steam, poach or bake fish. Don't deep fry it in batter – even in vegetable oil – since the batter absorbs a lot of the frying fat.

Use as little oil or fat as possible when cooking. Choose one that is low in saturates and high in monosaturates and polyunsaturates (see tables on pages 117 and 118). Sunflower, soya and corn oils are best, followed by olive oil. Place some olive oil on the table and encourage the family to develop a taste for it, especially on salads.

Avoid lard, coconut oil, palm oil, hard margarine, butter and ghee. Mixed vegetable oils can be very confusing and contain a lot more saturated fat than pure vegetable oil, so it is best to leave them well alone.

When *stir-frying* it is best to use a steep-sided, round-bottomed pan like a wok. These allow you to fry using a small amount of oil.

If you love chips and simply must have them, cut them thick and straight (so there is less surface area to soak up the oil or fat) and fry them in sunflower, soya or corn oil and drain off fat on kitchen paper. Use the oil only twice or three times before throwing it away (it will have become hydrogenated). It is now possible to buy oven-ready chips cooked in sunflower oil.

If you must fry use a non-stick pan and you might not have to add any fat or oil at all.

Convenience and fast foods

Convenience foods are not necessarily junk foods. Many are first class – for instance frozen peas, tinned beans and frozen fish. The problem arises with products such as pies, burgers, hot dogs, sausages, biscuits, chocolates, crisps and so on. It may be very difficult to know what is in a product such as pre-packed pizza unless it is stated on the packaging.

Take a few examples. In a food very popular with children, such as pizza, the saturated fat content will depend on what fat is used in baking the bread base, which cheeses are put on top and the quantity and type of meat, if any, that is included in the topping. It should be possible to make your own pizzas with relatively low-fat ingredients, but if you eat out or buy a pizza ready made then you must consider the fat content as part of your planned intake.

The Massachusetts Medical Society Committee on Nutrition looked into the amount of junk food eaten in the United States, and their results were published in the *New England Journal* in September 1989: 'Every second, an estimated two hundred people in the United States order one or more hamburgers.' On a typical day, one in five Americans eat at a fast food restaurant, of which there were 140,000 in 1980. Britain appears to be following the American lead. With hamburgers and hot dogs, as with sausages, assessing how much saturated fat you are eating is difficult but not impossible (see list below). Official definitions of meat content may be very misleading – for instance in sausages where a declaration of, say 60 per cent meat could result in a great deal of saturated fat being retained, because meat is defined as a minimum of 50 per cent lean. In pies there is extra fat in the pastry. If you eat a lot in this type of restaurant try changing to baked potatoes, salads and leaner meats or non-battered fish. Restaurants are, after all, acutely sensitive to what the public wants. It's up to us, the customers, to call the tune.

A general tip is to be suspicious of all so-called junk food. Inspect the labels for percentages of unsaturated fat and assume that the rest must be saturated. Many of the fast food restaurants in the UK are now following the American lead and declaring the fat content of their meals. This will certainly help you in working out your daily intake and should therefore be encouraged.

The following list is not comprehensive but includes many fast and convenience foods. Where we give the amount of fat for an item of food, rather than 100 g, we assume an average-sized portion. We are grateful to Wimpy and McDonalds for the information given on their meals.

Fat content of fast and convenience foods

Type of Food	Total fat (g) per item	Saturated fat (g) per item
Traditional UK foods		
Sausage roll	20 per 60 g roll	assume 10
Steak and kidney pie	42 per 200 g pie	assume 21
Pork pie	38 per 140 g pie	assume 19
Fruit pie with pastry	15.5	4.3
Fried fish in batter	20 for large fish	depends on cooking oil
Chips, fried	22 for chip-shop portion	depends on cooking oil
Black pudding	22 per 100 g	assume 50 per cent saturate
Mayonnaise	78.9 per 100 g	varies with oil
Yorkshire pudding	10.1	varies with cooking fat
Fried pork sausage	14.7	assume 7.3
Frankfurter (large)	12.5	assume 6.3
Toffee	17.2 per 100 g	assume 7 g
Chocolate	32 per 100 g	assume 18 g
Fast food restaurants		
Wimpy		
Hamburger	9.6	assume 4.8
Cheeseburger	13	assume 6.7
King-size Wimpy	20.6	assume 10.4
Quarter-pounder	30	assume 15
Half-pounder	51.4	assume 25.7
Bacon and egg in bun	23.4	assume 11.7
Milk shake	6.6	assume 6.4
McDonalds		
Hamburger	9.9	5.0
Cheeseburger	13.6	6.7
Quarter-pounder	19.3	9.1
Quarter-pounder + cheese	26.4	14
Fried fish	24.6	5.3
French fries (regular portion)	14.5	7.9
Chicken nuggets	16.4 per six	4.4 per six
Apple pie	15.4	4.3
Plain doughnut	16.3	7.6
Choc doughnut	19.5	10.2
Milk shake	6.1	4.3

The importance of fibre

Fibre is the background skeletal structure of many plants, such as cereals (wheat, oats, corn, etc.), most vegetables and most fruits. It also has another great advantage. None of the fibre in a food is lost through cooking.

The modern interest in fibre came from the realization that people in the Third World, who do not suffer 'Western diseases', eat much more fibre in their diets than us. We eat about 20 g a day whereas in Africa, for instance, they eat more than 100 g a day. This was believed an important contribution to the fact that on their native diet Africans do not suffer from irritable bowel syndrome, constipation, diverticular disease and possibly even large bowel cancer. They also have a lower incidence of dental decay and gallstones. More fibre in the diet may improve the control of diabetes, and can greatly help to reduce weight because food high in fibre tends to be filling in relatively small amounts. Increasing the amounts of fibre in your diet may also have additional benefits in preventing coronary heart disease.

Soluble and insoluble fibre

There are two types of fibre: water-soluble and water-insoluble. Most of what we recognize as high-fibre food contains water-insoluble fibre, for instance wheat bran. This is the type that helps prevent or control bowel complaints. Most of the fibre in oats and beans is water-soluble and this is the type that appears to be most promising in the control of heart disease. It is best taken in the form of oat bran or oatmeal, for instance in breakfast cereal or in bread or baking.

Fibre is obtained in meals that include beans, wholemeal bread, oatmeal bread and cakes, and wholemeal pasta. Adults should try to eat at least 30 g of fibre a day (about the same amount as saturated fat).

How to eat more fibre

Eat plenty of bread, best in thick slices. Choose wholemeal rather than white. Chapatis, hard dough and pitta bread are very good, provided they are made from wholemeal flour.

Use wholemeal flour instead of white flour for baking.

Choose the right breakfast cereal. Many of these are high in fibre as well as vitamins and iron.

Deliberately increase the amount of peas, beans and lentils you eat. Beans in particular may make the basis of a meal themselves. Tinned beans are just as good.

Eat more potatoes, which are an excellent source of energy as carbohydrate. Most of the fibre is, however, in the skin, so try baking them in their jackets. Sweet potatoes and yams are equally good sources of energy and fibre.

Brown rice is better than white. It may take a bit longer to cook, but doesn't stick to the same extent and tastes nicer.

Make a policy of putting out *unsalted* nuts and dried fruit and take these as mini-snacks instead of biscuits or chocolates. Be careful, however, about eating too many if you are trying to lose weight, since they contain quite a few calories.

Try to eat fruit and a good range of vegetables at least once a day. They not only contain a lot of fibre and are filling without containing too many calories, but they also contain very important vitamins.

How to read the nutritional content of food

Most supermarket foods now give nutritional information, and it is easily understood if you read the contents carefully. Somewhere on the packet, the can or the bottle you will find a list. For example, on a 450 g tin of Heinz baked beans the contents read:

Amount per 100 g	[note: a serving is about 225 g]
Fat	0.3 g
(of which saturates)	0.1 g
Protein	5.0 g
Carbohydrate	13.1 g
(of which sugars)	6.0 g
Energy	306 kJ/72 kcal
Sodium	0.5 g
Dietary fibre	7.3 g

Interpreting this should prove easy. There are 72 calories in every 100 g, or 162 calories per 225 g serving. Very little is fat, and only 0.1 g is saturated fat. Most of the calories clearly come from carbohydrate, of which roughly half is sugar. There is a great deal of fibre present, but whether soluble or insoluble is unspecified.

Carbohydrates

Once upon a time, slimming diets were low in carbohydrate and tended to include quite a lot of fat early in the day. Remember the old slogan: 'Eat fat to lose weight'? With better understanding we now prize complex carbohydrates as excellent sources of energy and vitamins, and they form an integral part of a balanced healthy diet.

The two commonest sources of complex carbohydrates are bread and potatoes. Apart from the calorie considerations, these are both very healthy and nutritious components of our diet and we use plenty of them in our recipes. With bread, choose a high-fibre type such as wholemeal or oatmeal. With potatoes, avoid roasting them and keep chips to once or twice a week, following tips already given about cooking them. Boiled potatoes are good, provided you don't melt butter over them. Baked are even better and very easy these days in a microwave. Try to eat the skin too: it is an excellent source of fibre. Flavour your jacket potatoes with low-fat cottage cheese or natural yogurt with chives.

Salt

Let's not get too carried away about salt. The majority of the population can cope very well with the 10 g or so we eat in our daily diet. But a minority cannot. These are people with a tendency to raised blood pressure, people with certain types of heart disease, liver disease and kidney disease. If you have raised blood pressure you will undoubtedly be under the care of your doctor, who will advise you on salt intake. People who already suffer from heart disease will also take sensible pre-cautions about salt. But this does not mean taking no salt at all. It is vital, and with no salt in our diet we would become very ill indeed. Most of us need only 1 g a day for our body's needs; we eat the other 9 g because we have developed a taste for it. Salt's only connection with heart attacks is its link with high blood pressure, which we deal with in Chapter 10.

Most of the salt we eat is put into our food at the processing, manufacturing and cooking stages: 75 per cent of our intake gets into our food in this way. Some comes in ready-bought food, more is added during cooking and only about 15–25 per cent is sprinkled on our food before eating it. If you would like some general tips about salt intake, here are some that might help.

Use less salt in cooking.

Use less in flavouring, or try other flavours such as

lemon juice, herbs, spices, pepper and mustard. Salt substitutes, obtained from the chemists, contain less than ordinary table salt but most still contain some salt. These are not necessary at all for the average person's diet. Sea salt has other minerals in it but is no better than table salt in its general salt content.

Cut down on salty snacks such as crisps and salted nuts.

If you buy tinned vegetables, buy the ones marked 'no added salt'.

Cut down on ready-salted meats and fish such as bacon, gammon, salt beef and salt mackerel.

Use fewer tinned and packet soups. A single serving can contain 1–3 g of salt. Make your own soups instead.

Putting all the dietary advice into practice

We have given a lot of information in this chapter. The advice on fish is simple and is the most important new message of this book. But it should be taken as part of a dietary package, together with our advice on saturated and unsaturated fat intake, fibre and salt. To give you a broader idea of how to bring all this together, at the end of Chapter 9 we have drawn up a week's sample menu with practical examples of how to eat healthily day by day.

Of course it's difficult to change your eating habits – we recognize that. But with the right will and a sense of purpose you can get round any obstacle course. You won't go far wrong if you couple understanding with a sense of humour and allow your natural common sense to prevail.

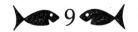

9

Recipes for a Healthy Heart

RECIPES FOR OILY FISH

Tuna and smoked mackerel pâté

Pâtés need a fatty binding agent, such as butter. This dish offers the low saturated fat alternative, skimmed milk, while retaining all of a pâté's texture and flavour.

    1 × 210 g/7½ oz can tuna in brine
    250 g/8 oz smoked mackerel fillet
    1 slice white bread, crusts removed and cubed
    2–3 tablespoons skimmed milk
    1 tablespoon lemon juice
    grated rind of 1 lemon

Drain the tuna. Remove the skin and bones from the mackerel and flake it. Blend all the ingredients in a food processor if you have one, otherwise mash them thoroughly with a fork. Chill and serve with wholemeal toast, crusty brown rolls and a salad.

Mackerel Portuguese

Notice in this dish that we have avoided high-fat creamy or buttery sauces, while including the beneficial mono-unsaturate, olive oil. Garlic too is now believed to be beneficial!

Serves 4

   4 mackerel, cleaned
   salt *and* pepper to taste

for the sauce:
   1 tablespoon olive oil
   ½ small onion
   1 clove garlic, crushed
   1 red or green pepper
   350 g/12 oz tomatoes, skinned, deseeded and chopped
   1 teaspoon paprika

to serve
   1 lemon
   chopped parsley

Preheat the oven to 350°F/180°C/gas mark 4. Split and bone the mackerel (it is best to ask your fishmonger to do this for you). Wash and dry them well. Place them in an ovenproof dish, season, and squeeze a little lemon juice over them. Bake for 20–25 minutes. Heat the olive oil and soften the onion in it. Add the garlic, pepper, tomatoes and paprika, while simmering very slowly and stirring often until the mixture is pulpy. Spoon this over the fish and serve with lemon quarters and chopped parsley.

Grilled salmon steak

This is a very savoury and full-bodied dish, yet easy and very quick to prepare.

Serves 4

   4 salmon steaks
   1 teaspoon sunflower oil
   lemon juice

Grease a piece of aluminium foil with sunflower oil. Place the salmon steaks on the foil and transfer them to the grill pan. Grill for about 5 minutes each side. Serve with boiled or mashed potatoes and a mixed salad. (Resist the temptation to spread the butter over the potatoes. Choose a moist vegetable instead of the salad, or mix skimmed milk with the potatoes.)

Halibut with mushrooms

Filling and easy to prepare, this is a delight when cooked in a little of your favourite cider.

Serves 4

    180 g/6 oz mushrooms, peeled and chopped
    1 onion, finely chopped
    4 halibut steaks
    1 egg, beaten
    3 tablespoons breadcrumbs
    1 tablespoon lemon juice
    salt *and* pepper
    4 tablespoons cider

Preheat the oven to 325°F/170°C/gas mark 3. Place the mushrooms and onion in an ovenproof dish. Dip the halibut steaks in egg and coat with breadcrumbs. Place them on top of the onion and mushrooms, sprinkle with a little lemon juice and add salt and pepper sparingly. Pour the cider over the top. Bake for 40–50 minutes until tender. Serve with new potatoes and carrots.

Trout with almonds

Trout is a favourite fish for many people and it is also very good for you. Try not to buy trout harvested on a farm that uses soybean or vegetable feeds. Your fishmonger may be able to advise you about this.

Serves 4

> 4 trout, cleaned, washed and dried
> 60 g/2 oz flaked almonds
> salt *and* pepper
> 1 lemon

Place trout on aluminium foil and grill for 3–4 minutes each side. Sprinkle the fish with the almonds and put them back under the grill to brown. Season, and serve with lemon quarters.

For potatoes, choose boiled rather than chips. Use vegetables you like but avoid putting butter on them. An alternative would be to serve the trout with boiled rice, adding a small can of sweet corn and peppers – when cooked, sprinkle the rice with a little soya sauce. (Note that sauces such as soya, HP and so on contain a lot of salt, so you will not need to sprinkle salt on the fish as well.)

Tuna fish salad with baked potatoes

A great dish for summer weather, and one of the quickest to prepare for people who are in a hurry.

Serves 4

> 1 × 210 g/7½ oz can tuna in brine
> 1 cooking apple, peeled, cored and diced
> 2 boiled potatoes, diced
> 2 sticks celery, diced
> 1 small can beetroot (about 200 g/7 oz) or ½ jar whole small
>   beetroots, diced
> 1 small can peas (about 150 g/5 oz) *or* small packet frozen
>   peas

Drain the tuna, put it into a bowl and flake it with a fork. Add the apple and potato to the tuna. Prepare the dressing as follows:

3 tablespoons salad cream (choose reduced fat)
2 tablespoons plain yogurt
salt *and* pepper
sugar to taste
1 small clove garlic, crushed (optional)

Mix the salad cream and yogurt together, season with a little salt and pepper (and, if you like, sugar) and the garlic, if included.

Pour the dressing over the mixture in the bowl and mix carefully with a fork. Turn the salad into a serving dish and add the celery, beetroot and peas. Surround with crisp lettuce or watercress and tomato slices.

Fish curry

This illustrates how you can replace meat in a fairly common recipe and still enjoy the same flavours.

Serves 4

2 tablespoons olive oil
1 onion, chopped
½ green pepper
1 carrot, thinly sliced
1 tablespoon curry powder
flour
1 teaspoon lemon juice
300 ml/½ pint fish stock
1 apple, peeled, cored and chopped
1 tablespoon sultanas
500 g/1 oz haddock
salt *and* pepper
chopped parsley

Melt the margarine in a pan and fry the onion, pepper, carrot and curry powder for 5 minutes. Stir in the flour and cook for 1 minute. Gradually stir in the lemon juice and stock. Heat, stirring, until the sauce thickens. Add the chopped apple, sultanas and fish, then season to taste with salt and pepper. Cover, and simmer for about 20–25 minutes.

Put on to a hot serving dish and garnish with chopped parsley. Serve with brown rice, sliced tomato, diced cucumber and natural yogurt.

Grilled mackerel with gooseberry sauce

Why not experiment with this blending of fruity flavours and the savoury taste of fish!

Serves 4

> 4 mackerel, filleted
> 250 g/8 oz gooseberries
> sugar *or* honey to taste

Trim and clean the mackerel fillets. Cook on a piece of foil under a medium grill. Meanwhile poach the gooseberries with a little water and sugar or honey to taste. When soft, rub the gooseberries through a sieve, or liquidize them in a blender, return the purée to the pan and reheat. Serve the mackerel with the sauce and add grilled tomatoes and vegetables.

Cod baked with vegetables

Cod is not an oily fish, but this meal would make a delicious alternative to one of the meat or poultry dishes on your non oily-fish days. Note the olive oil which is high in monounsaturates. Top-quality virgin olive oil will give the best results.

Serves 4

    4 cod steaks
    1 tablespoon lemon juice
    freshly ground black pepper
    1 tablespoon olive oil
    1 small onion, finely chopped
    1 small green pepper, deseeded and sliced
    3 sticks celery, chopped
    6 tomatoes, skinned and chopped
    1 clove garlic (optional)
    a little salt
    ½ teaspoon oregano
    250 g/8 oz button mushrooms, sliced

Preheat the oven to 350°F/180°C/gas mark 4. Wash and dry the steaks and place them in a shallow ovenproof dish. Sprinkle with the lemon juice and freshly ground black pepper. Heat the olive oil in a pan and lightly fry the onion, green pepper and celery. Add the tomatoes, garlic, salt and oregano. Bring to the boil and simmer for 10 minutes. Add the mushrooms and simmer for a further 5 minutes. Pour the vegetables over the fish, cover with foil and cook for 30–40 minutes.

Grilled fresh sardines with salad

An excellent and quick lunchtime snack. Allow three sardines per person, or more according to appetite. Grill over foil, with no added butter or margarine, and serve with a side salad and wholemeal bread.

RECIPES LOW IN SATURATES

Paella

Low in saturated fat yet deliciously savoury, colourful and economical, paella is quick and easy to make.

Remember that the fat in chicken is attached to the skin, so remove the skin before cooking. Note also that this recipe contains shellfish, which many people think are forbidden because of their cholesterol content. We believe this to be an exaggeration. Modern analysis has suggested that most shellfish usually contain much the same level of cholesterol as other animal produce, such as lean red meat. The quantities per person are also very low.

Serves 4

  2 tablespoons olive oil
  1 medium Spanish onion, chopped
  ½ red pepper, diced
  ½ green pepper, diced
  2 chicken breasts, cut into chunks
  750 ml/1¼ pints boiling water
  1 chicken stock cube
  ½ teaspoon turmeric
  salt *and* pepper
  350 g/12 oz easy-cook American rice
  90 g/3 oz frozen peas
  125 g/4 oz prawns
  8 mussels, cooked

Heat the oil in a large saucepan and add the chopped onion and peppers. Cook over low heat until slightly softened. Add the chicken and cook for 5 minutes, stirring regularly. Pour in 600 ml/1 pint of the boiling water, the stock cube, turmeric, salt and pepper. Add the rice and bring to the boil. Stir with a fork to separate the grains and simmer, uncovered, for 10 minutes. Then add the peas and prawns and continue cooking until the rice is tender and the liquid absorbed. It may be necessary to add more liquid, as this dish is not intended to be too dry. Add the mussels 2–3 minutes before the rice is cooked, and cover to heat through.

Chicken fricassee

Another poultry dish, this is low in saturated fat and makes good family eating. Note that the milk used is skimmed.

1 × 1.75 kg/3½ lb chicken, jointed and skinned
1 large onion, chopped
2–3 medium carrots, thinly sliced
1 head of celery, cut into chunks
1 tablespoon dried thyme *or* about 3 fresh sprigs if available
2 bayleaves
600–900 ml/1–1½ pints skimmed milk (the sauce is intended to be light)
salt *and* pepper
1 level tablespoon cornflour, blended with a little milk

Preheat the oven to 350°F/180°C/gas mark 4. Place the chicken pieces in a large casserole dish. Add the chopped onion, carrots, celery, thyme, bayleaves, milk, and salt and pepper. Cover with a tightly fitting lid and cook for 1½ hours or until the chicken is done. Stir in the cornflour and return the dish to the oven for 15 minutes.

This dish is better made the day before and left in the refrigerator overnight. Serve with plain boiled potatoes.

Chilli con carne

Choose a piece of lean meat and either get the butcher to mince it or do so yourself. Mixing the meat with beans means that much less meat is eaten and therefore less saturated fat. An additional benefit is the high fibre content of the beans.

Serves 4

350 g/12 oz lean minced beef
1 beef stock cube
1 medium onion, chopped

1 x 397 g/14 oz tin chopped tomatoes
¼ teaspoon ground cumin
2 teaspoons vinegar
1 teaspoon sugar
¼–½ level teaspoon chilli powder
1 x 397 g/14 oz tin red kidney beans in chilli sauce
salt *and* pepper to taste
1 tablespoon tomato purée

Dry-fry the mince in a heavy-bottomed frying pan until browned. Cover with water and bring to the boil, simmer for 5 minutes, then transfer the mixture to a heat-resistant bowl. There are now two ways of removing the fat. You can prepare the mince the day before, let it stand overnight and spoon off the solidified fat next day. Alternatively, if you cover the mince in cold water, allow it to cool to room temperature before placing it in the refrigerator, this will again solidify the fat, which can then be lifted off. You should not put hot mince in your fridge since it will raise the temperature inside the fridge, creating a problem with hygiene.

Transfer the skimmed meat and stock to a saucepan and add the onion, tomatoes, cumin, vinegar, sugar, stock cube, and chilli powder. Simmer for about 1 hour, making sure it doesn't get too dry. Add the chilli beans, salt and pepper and tomato purée before cooking for a further 15 minutes. Serve with boiled rice.

Chicken with peppers

Virtually free of saturated fat, this is a nourishing and very appetizing meat dish.

Serves 4

4 chicken breasts
1 tablespoon olive oil
½ small onion, sliced
4 tomatoes, chopped

1 green pepper, deseeded and sliced
2 red peppers
1 clove garlic, crushed
pinch dried thyme
pinch chilli powder
150 ml/¼ pint dry white wine
salt *and* pepper

Preheat the oven to 350°F/180°C/gas mark 4. Remove the skin from chicken breasts and place them in a large ovenproof dish that has a closely fitting lid. Heat the olive oil and add the onion, tomatoes, peppers, garlic, thyme and chilli powder. Cook until slightly softened, turning frequently. Add to the chicken. Now pour the wine over the chicken and season with pepper and just a little salt. Cover the dish and bake for 1–1½ hours, until the chicken is tender and the vegetables are soft.

Serve with baked or boiled potatoes and vegetables. (Note that this freezes well. It is a good idea therefore to make a double quantity, using 300 ml/½ pint of dry white wine.)

Spaghetti Bolognese

Here is another meat dish with relatively small quantities of saturated fat per person. Choose a wholemeal spaghetti.

Serves 4

350 g/12 oz lean mince
1 large onion, chopped
1 x 397 g/14 oz tin chopped tomatoes
1 clove garlic, crushed (optional)
1 bayleaf
1 tablespoon Italian seasoning, according to taste
1 teaspoon oregano
salt *and* pepper
tomato purée to thicken

Dry-fry the mince (see instructions in the chilli con carne recipe on page 149), turning until browned. Cover the meat with cold water, bring to the boil and simmer for 5 minutes before transferring to a heatproof dish and allowing to cool to room temperature. Place in the fridge and, when cold, skim the fat off the surface and drain off the surplus water.

Return the mince to the pan and add the chopped onion, tomatoes, garlic, bay leaf, herbs, and salt and pepper to taste. Cover, and cook slowly for about 1 hour, taking care not to let the mixture boil dry. Stir in the tomato purée until the desired consistency is reached. Serve with wholemeal spaghetti.

Luxury ratatouille

A vegetarian delight, and probably the best ratatouille you have ever tasted! Not only does it contain little saturated fat, but it includes two ingredients now believed to protect against heart attacks – olive oil and garlic.

Serves 8 (but half can be frozen)

    500 g/1 lb aubergines, chopped
    500 g/1 lb courgettes, sliced
    2–3 tablespoons seasoned flour
    olive oil for frying – pick the best quality
    1 bottle fruity white wine (Chardonnay is a good one)
    250 g/8 oz red peppers, coarsely chopped
    250 g/8 oz green peppers, coarsely chopped
    500 g/1 lb onions
    500 g/1 lb tomatoes *or* 1 x 397 g/14 oz tin
    4 cloves garlic, crushed
    2 teaspoons sugar
    1 sprig fresh basil *or* 1 teaspoon dried
    1 tablespoon tomato purée
    salt *and* pepper

Chop the vegetables and keep separate. Sprinkle the aubergines and courgettes with the seasoned flour. Heat some olive oil in a frying pan and add the aubergines. When softened slightly, transfer it to a large pan. This will leave some seasoned flour in the pan. Add 150 ml/ ¼ pint of the wine to the frying pan and stir well to incorporate the floury juices. Pour this on to the aubergines. Repeat the process with the courgettes.

Then add some more olive oil to the pan and fry the peppers and onions; when softened add them to the other vegetables. Place the tomatoes, garlic, sugar, basil and tomato purée in a separate pan, add a little salt and pepper and simmer for a few minutes to reduce the liquid slightly. Rub this through a sieve or liquidize briefly to give a fairly thick tomato sauce and add it to the other ingredients. Pour in the rest of the wine and cook on top of the stove until the vegetables are cooked but not mushy.

Spoon off the olive oil, which will lie on the surface of the ratatouille. Serve with boiled white rice (the vegetables provide sufficient fibre and the colour contrast is beautiful).

If cooking for only 4, interrupt the cooking while the vegetables are still firm, take half the mixture, cool it and then freeze it. Carry on cooking the remainder. The frozen portion can be cooked to completion at a later date.

The alternative Sunday joint

Why not alternate Sunday roasts between traditional meats such as beef, lamb and pork, and low saturated fat poultry such a chicken and turkey? Or with a lovely dish of baked salmon?

Roast turkey with stuffing

Serves a family (with meat for sandwiches during the week)

Place the turkey in a roasting tin and spread a little high polyunsaturate fat over the breast and legs. Cover with foil and cook according to your oven instructions.

While the turkey is cooking, chill a little water in a large Pyrex jug in the fridge. When the turkey is cooked, pour the juices into the chilled water and place in the coldest part of your fridge until the fat starts to solidify on top. Skim this off and use some of the remaining turkey stock in the stuffing and some to make the gravy.

To make the stuffing first chop an onion finely. Place it in a non-stick pan, cover with water and boil until soft. Add 90 g/3 oz Paxo sage and onion (which contains just 2 g saturated fat) and simmer for a few minutes, adding turkey stock and enough water to ensure it doesn't become too dry.

Serve with boiled potatoes and two vegetables of your choice.

Finally, here's a delicious, attractive, low-fat pudding.

Strawberry fluff

Serves 1

   1 teaspoon gelatine
   2 teaspoons hot water
   a little grated orange peel
   1 x 150 g/5 oz tub low-fat strawberry yogurt
   1 egg white
   pinch salt

Warm a cup by putting in into a saucepan of simmering water. Dissolve the gelatine in the 2 teaspoons of hot water in the cup, which should be still in the simmering water. Stir until the gelatine has dissolved. Now add the orange peel to the strawberry yogurt and stir to mix. Add a little of this mixture to the simmering cup. Then tip the cup's contents into the rest of the cold yogurt, stirring briskly until well mixed. Leave until it begins to set. Timing is important. At this stage, whisk the egg white (from a salmonella-free source, these days) with the salt until it starts to thicken and begins to firm. Now fold it into the strawberry mixture and mix gently before spooning into a serving dish. Place in the fridge until it has set.

SEVEN-DAY SAMPLE MENU

This menu gives average portions, but these can be varied according to the appetites and calorie needs of readers and their families. Our aim is health rather than weight reduction, although a healthy diet will usually keep you to a healthy weight. But a hard-working manual labourer will need vastly more calories in his diet than a lightly built woman working in a centrally heated office.

We have tried to include as wide-ranging and interesting a range of items as possible. We also provide more than the minimum of 30 g/1 oz a week of oily fish; the ingredients of the menu should make the intake of less than 30 g/1 oz per day of saturated fat as effortless as possible.

We would advise you to drink about four or five cups of normal tea or coffee per day (it is not necessary to buy decaffeinated if you don't drink more than this amount in a day) and to make any further liquid intake either cold fruit juice, or fruit squash with boiling water added.

Monday

Breakfast
Porridge, made with water. Sweeten with honey or a few sultanas and pour a little skimmed milk over it. A slice wholemeal toast, with marmalade or a light covering of polyunsaturated margarine or low-fat spread. If it must be real butter, measure what you usually put on your knife and work out the saturated fat so that you include it in your daily 30 g/1 oz. Try a hot orange drink instead of tea or coffee.

Lunch
Tuna sandwiches, again with wholemeal or a high-fibre bread, followed by fresh fruit or a low-fat yogurt. Remember that a small lunch allows you to participate in a larger family meal in the evening. If your main meal is at lunchtime, then reverse these two meals. Cup of tea with skimmed or semi-skimmed milk. (Note: if you want full-cream milk, keep the quantity to a minimum of milk and add the saturated fat content to your daily total. One full bottle of full-cream milk is more than two-thirds of your advised total daily saturated fat.)

Dinner
150 g/5 oz grilled steak per person with a mixed salad and one or two baked potatoes. Be careful with the salad cream and dressings: choose one that is low in saturated fat, which usually tastes just as pleasant. Don't be tempted to stuff the baked potato with butter. Use low-fat cottage cheese or, better still, experiment with your own dressings using natural yogurt with mint and cucumber, which is quite delicious. Have a single glass of red wine with it.

There is no need to deny that liking for sweet things. Core a medium cooking apple, and stuff it with about 30 g/1 oz of sultanas and 2 teaspoons of water. Prick the skin to stop it bursting and then microwave it for 2½ minutes on high power. Cover with foil immediately and leave to stand for a few minutes – it continues to bake, and this also avoids the danger of burning your mouth. Serve with a tablespoon of low-fat ice cream. Follow this with a beverage of your choice.

Snack
What about those little gastronomic cravings late at night? Watch the calories of course, but try a slice of wholemeal toast with delicious low-fat tuna and mackerel pâté (recipe on page 141).

Tuesday

Breakfast
As Monday, or try the alternative – fresh grapefruit or grapefruit tinned in its own juices, followed by either your favourite cereal (containing plenty of iron) and a thin slice of wholemeal toast with honey. Cup of coffee.

Lunch
Turkey breast sandwiches with wholemeal bread. Spread the slices only very lightly with high polyunsaturated margarine. This is made much easier if the margarine has been kept at room temperature long enough to soften. If you use a moister filling than turkey, such as tinned tuna or mackerel pâté, you will need no spread at all. Follow with fresh fruit or low-fat yogurt, and a cup of hot fruit juice.

Dinner
Grilled trout with almonds and mashed potatoes (see recipe on page 143). Remember to use skimmed milk with the potatoes rather than butter. Serve with lashings of soft grilled tomatoes and peas. Optional – one small glass of white wine.

Follow with a meringue nest filled with fresh fruit, topped with low-fat fruit yogurt or fromage frais. Beverage of your choice.

Snack

For a night-time (or elevenses) snack, take 2 Ryvita with cottage cheese, topped with a quartered tomato and a couple of slices of cucumber and seasoned with freshly ground black pepper. Avoid tea or coffee late at night because of the caffeine content. Try squash with boiling water instead.

Wednesday

Breakfast

Fruit juice followed by 2 Weetabix sweetened with sultanas and with hot skimmed milk poured over. Cup of tea.

Lunch

A low-fat cheese such as Edam, with lettuce, cucumber and spring onion. As an alternative to cheese consider a slice or two of lean ham or lean beef (not corned beef). Another alternative is tinned sardines or pilchards in tomato sauce, mashed on an unbuttered thick slice of wholemeal bread, then grilled. Follow with a cup of coffee.

Dinner

Chicken with peppers (see recipe on page 150), served with new or boiled potatoes and vegetables such as broccoli and carrots.

Follow this with strawberry fluff (see recipe on page 154) and a beverage of your choice.

Snack

Breakfast cereal, half portion, with hot or cold skimmed milk. Hot fruit juice.

Thursday

Breakfast
Kippers with a slice of wholemeal toast, followed by a refreshing glass of chilled fresh fruit juice. Note that frozen packaged kippers often arrive with butter in the bag. Either buy your kippers fresh or remove them from the pack, take out the butter and then poach or grill them. Follow it up with a cup of tea with skimmed milk.

Lunch
Baked beans on toast followed by mixed fruit salad, topped, if you like, with natural yogurt. Cup of tea.

Dinner
Paella (see recipe on page 147), followed by fruit jelly with real fruit, such as unsweetened pineapple and natural yogurt topping. (Low-fat ice cream would also go with jelly or fruit salads.)

Snack
Slice of hot wholemeal toast with your favourite jam, or two low-fat biscuits.

Friday

Breakfast
Fresh unsweetened fruit juice. Boiled or poached egg with wholemeal toast.

Lunch
Cold roast chicken or turkey breast with potatoes, salad and wholemeal bread. Cup of tea or coffee.

Dinner
Grilled mackerel with gooseberry sauce (see recipe on page 146). Serve with boiled potatoes and vegetables.

One of the best ways of cooking vegetables is in the pressure cooker or the microwave. Aim to get your moisture with the meal from the vegetables rather than from a buttery or creamy sauce. Follow this with stewed apple (or other fruit of your choice) and a small portion of low-fat ice cream.

Snack
Banana.

Saturday

Breakfast
Cereal with skimmed milk and sultanas. Slice of whole-meal toast with honey or marmalade.

Lunch
Lean ham sandwiches with mustard – or even better still, if your purse will run to it, smoked salmon or smoked trout sandwiches – and a side salad or low-calorie coleslaw.

Dinner
Ratatouille with white rice (see recipe on page 152). For a sweet here's another little treat – raspberry surprise! Into a small glass bowl put 4 raspberries, then 4 dessert-spoons of low-fat yogurt and 1 teaspoon runny honey. Cap with a plentiful helping of raspberries.

Snack
A couple of morning coffee biscuits.

Sunday

Breakfast
If the dinner is to be a red meat roast, why not start the day with grilled kippers, which will counter the blood

fat effects of the main meal. Put the kippers directly on to dry wholemeal toast – the oil in the kippers is moist enough to make up for butter or margarine.

Lunch

Roast beef (try to alternate this one week in three with roast chicken or turkey or baked salmon). Choose a lean cut of meat and don't eat any obvious fat or add cooking fat. Serve with baked potatoes and two vegetables, steamed in the pressure cooker or cooked in the microwave. If you like gravy, choose a mix such as Bisto, which does not have added fat. Bisto contains its own salt so you do not need to add any. Avoid the strong temptation to make your own gravy with the meat juices, since this will add a lot of saturated fat. With practice and experiment you will discover other techniques of making sauces, particularly vegetable and olive oil-based ones, that are really delicious, go well with boiled and mashed potatoes, and do not contain much saturated fat. After the main course treat yourself to home-baked apple pie, but try to cut back on the pastry and be sure to use only polyunsaturated margarine. You could allow yourself a little single cream on this one day – alternatively low-fat ice cream or natural yogurt.

Dinner

Low-fat cheese with crispbread and half a 450 g/15 oz can of low-fat rice pudding. Instead of jam, put a few strawberry halves in the middle.

Snack

If turkey or salmon was the main meal, a little of this in a wholemeal sandwich.

10

Lifestyles

For a very long time there has been reluctance on the part of both the medical profession and the public to consider preventive health measures. This certainly does not arise from logic, since we are all well aware that prevention is far better than cure. It arises for a number of more subtle reasons.

Prevention implies a different philosophy towards living and eating patterns, and the willpower to continue this effort not for a few weeks or even months but for life. This is difficult. The medical profession, while well aware of the benefits of prevention, is so over-worked with treating diseases that it cannot find enough time for truly preventive measures. It isn't that doctors don't care – what they need is help from an informed and willing public.

The last decade has seen a revolution in the desire of ordinary people to understand medical matters – consider the space devoted to health in women's magazines or the many medical programmes on television. These changes are for the best, and the relationship between the public and the caring professions as a whole, including nurses, dieticians and so on, must be developed and extended. But for the public to be able to help in the task of prevention, basic knowledge and understanding are needed. That has been the aim of this book.

We have shown how diet is a vital component in the risk factors that cause heart attacks; from the evidence of studies worldwide, diet is almost certainly *the* most important factor. We have discussed the vital importance of fish and fish oil in our daily diet. And we have looked carefully at other important elements of food, such as saturated fat intake.

But there are other very important risk factors that can often be readily eliminated. With a disease that is as common and as deadly as heart attack, we owe it to ourselves and our families to cut every risk factor known to science. Those others are all either acquired as habits, such as smoking, or forced upon us as part of our lifestyles, such as stress.

You really can quit smoking

Do non-smokers suffer heart attacks? The answer, most definitely, is Yes. Do smokers live to a grand old age without suffering heart attacks? The answer again is most definitely Yes. Therefore smoking cannot be a cause of heart attacks. But the answer to this is most definitely No – this is a false analogy. It's like saying: I cross the road every day, therefore people never die crossing the road. Smoking is very definitely one of the major causative factors of heart attacks.

Many people who recognize that smoking is a bad habit still choose to smoke. That is their right. We are all for freedom of choice, provided it does not interfere with others; but it is a sad fact that for many smoking is an addiction, and the real reason these people don't stop smoking is they *cannot*. Don't underestimate this difficulty. In a study performed many years ago on heroin addicts in Britain, more addicts managed to give up heroin than gave up smoking. Another large group of smokers say that they could give up, or at the very least cut down considerably, if it could be definitively proved to them that smoking does cause serious diseases such as heart attacks.

So we have two aims. First we shall very briefly outline the evidence against smoking. Secondly we shall give some helpful advice to smokers who really would like to kick the habit.

The evidence against smoking

There is irrefutable evidence that smoking causes the majority of cases of lung cancer. A heavy smoker, for instance a man or woman who smokes more than twenty cigarettes a day, has more than twenty times a non-smoker's risk of getting lung cancer. In Sheffield, with a population of roughly half a million, seven hundred people die each year from lung cancer. It is a very unpleasant disease and only 5 per cent of sufferers are still alive five years after its onset. In the same city, two thousand people a year die from coronary heart disease. Assuming that 20 per cent die in each heart attack, this would multiply to a staggering ten thousand people a year in Sheffield alone suffering either a heart attack or one of the very serious related complications. No wonder heart attack is by far the commonest serious acute medical emergency.

The link between smoking and heart attacks is just as powerful and well documented. Smoking has a number of damaging effects on the heart. The nicotine which is absorbed into your blood through the surface of the lungs is responsible for smoking being addictive, since it has chemical effects in your brain which lead to the 'need' to continue to smoke.

Nicotine narrows blood vessels. Studies have demonstrated that during the smoking of a single cigarette, those already narrowed coronary arteries actually narrow further still, making you more prone to angina and even increasing the risk of a fatal clot within the narrowed artery. In people with narrowed arteries to their legs (medically termed intermittent claudication), giving up smoking may make all the difference to avoiding high-risk operations or even amputation.

How many smokers realize that when they inhale they are taking highly poisonous carbon monoxide into their blood streams. Even in tiny doses, this clings much harder to the blood than does oxygen. As a result, even less oxygen gets carried through the narrowed arteries into the hard-working muscle of our heart wall. The results can be disastrous.

But it doesn't even stop there. In addition to the cancer-inducing tars contained in cigarette smoke, there are other factors that damage the lining of blood vessels, increasing the tendency to form that dreadful clogging atheroma. Smoking also lowers the beneficial HDL-cholesterol, as has been shown in many large medical trials. And, finally, to make matters even worse, smoking increases the tendency of platelets to stick to one another, bringing that fatal clot closer. You will not be surprised, therefore, to hear that medical trials the world over report little disagreement when they study smoking in relation to heart attacks.

One big study in the UK showed that men under the age of forty-five who smoked twenty-five or more cigarettes a day had fifteen times the risk of a heart attack compared to men of the same age who did not smoke. This difference was still present in much older men, but it became less pronounced, with men over forty-five running three times the risk if they smoked this quantity of cigarettes. These results have been confirmed in numerous studies all over the world.

But it doesn't just affect men. The appalling truth is that each year, in Britain alone, forty thousand women die from the effects of smoking. Can we really accept this terrible statistic? If a pill prescribed by doctors caused forty deaths a year, never mind forty thousand, it would immediately be taken off the market and the manufacturers would be sued.

Young women who smoke during pregnancy have smaller babies, which get a poorer start in life. And young women tend to be taking the pill, another risk factor.

What about pipe and cigar smoking?
The risk of a heart attack appears to be less than with cigarettes, but there is still an increased risk – and added to that there is a big increase in the risk of cancer of the tongue, throat and nose.

Good news too
If you give up smoking, your increased risk of a heart attack reduces very rapidly. If you need something to help you quit the habit, surely this great potential benefit is the best incentive.

How do I give up smoking?
For many people it is surprisingly easy. For instance, many of the thousands of patients we have seen with heart attacks give up smoking immediately – the shock frightens them into it. But how much more beneficial it would have been if they had given up before the heart attack and possibly avoided having it altogether!

It has been proved time and time again that even the most hardened smokers can throw out this disastrous habit.

There is no one simple way to give up smoking. What you need more than anything else is a strong reason –

such as avoiding heart attack and lung cancer – and a strong will to put it into effect. Some people are much more hooked than others. In general, the more cigarettes you smoke, the greater your dependency. But even if you have tried already and failed, this is no reason to give up. Most people make many attempts before they finally give up.

Some people worry that they will gain weight – this may be true, but it isn't due to a chemical in cigarettes that keeps your weight down. What happens when you smoke is that you damage your taste buds and so your appetite decreases; when you give it up, your taste and then your appetite improve. Obviously it must be possible to prevent weight gain by controlling your diet. The easiest way to achieve this is by eating more fruit and vegetables or any food that contains few calories and a lot of fibre. The list of high-fibre foods in Chapter 8 will help you. But remember that the battle to give up smoking is fought and won – or lost – in your own mind.

Here are some tips that might help you to throw away the habit:

Get your strong reason clear in your mind, so you know why you are doing it. Be prepared for friends and relatives to make fun of your resolve. Your own inner strength will come from the knowledge of how much good you will be doing yourself by the act of stopping. It is for yourself that you are giving up; only you yourself can do it. And remember that if another smoker makes a great joke of it, then he or she is probably consumed by envy at the prospect of your succeeding. Expect this person to tempt you with an opened pack or, worse still, by smoking provocatively in front of you.

Pick a time when it will be easiest to begin stopping. Don't try to give up at a time of maximum stress. If the family are all on top of you or your boss is making your life miserable at work, choose a time when you can get away from these stresses if that is possible. A good time to start might well be a week's holiday, whether spent at home or away, provided you can control your environment.

It takes about ten days before you can feel you are winning the battle. During those critical first ten days in particular avoid the sort of environment that is most conducive to smoking – pubs, parties, or a friend who is himself or herself a heavy smoker and will not like your giving it up. A far better solution would be to persuade your friend to join you in kicking the habit. That way you should achieve a kind of group therapy.

Ignore the persuasive arguments of those who don't want you to stop. Think about it and analyse their reasons. For example, consider that old chestnut of somebody remarking that their mother or father smoked and lived to be seventy-five. Nobody ever points to all the mothers and fathers who are not around to tell you that they smoked and did not live to be fifty.

There will be side-effects, particularly during those first few days, so be prepared for them. Recognize them for what they are. Don't exaggerate them. Before you start set up a routine that you'll follow when the side-effects disturb you. For instance, if you get irritable and jittery, do something physical that involves concentration so it takes your mind off both the cigarettes and your symptoms. Remember that after a few more days it will all be a thing of the past. We have found it helps patients to put the cost of cigarettes not smoked into a collection box and use it for something you really want, for instance a new item of clothing, something for the house, the garden, the kitchen – even an extra little holiday. That way you both gain the treat and realize just how much money you are saving.

Nicotine gum is only available on prescription, because nicotine is a potentially dangerous drug which itself can be addictive. Chewing the gum takes away some of the unpleasant mental and physical symptoms of withdrawal. Nicotine-based lozenges, which can be bought over the chemist's counter, have the same drawbacks.

There are plastic cigarettes called PAX which may help. You don't light them up, you merely draw on them and inhale a menthol-flavoured vapour, which makes some people feel easier during this difficult period. Others try harmless herbal remedies, such as chewing sunflower seeds or eating nuts. If you do this you need just to keep an eye on the calories, and if you chew nuts, choose unsalted. There are many alternative measures, including relaxation therapy, hypnosis and acupuncture. These appear to cause few or no side-effects, and if they help a really hardened smoker give up the habit they are worth it. Some advice on relaxation therapy appears later in this chapter.

Exercise

Once you have given up smoking it is relatively easy to continue as a non-smoker. With exercise, however, you have to devote both time and willpower for the rest of your life. Attitude is the most important thing. If you regard the exercise you need as corporal punishment, then you will not continue with it – no more should you. If you regard it as fun and invigorating, then you very likely will. Before you come to any conclusion, let's first look at the most up-to-date opinion on the value of exercise.

We all know that when we are physically fit and exercising regularly we *feel* better. There is no doubt that people who exercise regularly tend to have lower weights, less fat, less tachycardia (fast heart rate) in response to exercise, and to be fitter generally for all the demands of the modern long working day. But we have all heard of joggers who die from heart attacks out on the roads and in the parks. So does exercise really do our hearts any good?

The answer is probably Yes. But it has to be regular and you have to do enough of it.

The meaning of 'aerobics'

We have all heard the term 'aerobics' used in relation to exercise, but what does it mean? If you really sprint hard you tire quickly, and at the end you will find yourself very much out of breath with your heart pumping uncomfortably fast in your chest. What you have done is to exercise too fast for the oxygen arriving at your muscles. The muscles have gone on contracting hard even without oxygen, but you pay for it when you stop. This is called 'anaerobic' exercise and is clearly very heavy indeed. If, on the other hand, you exercise more lightly – by taking a brisk walk or a light run or jog – then the oxygen can arrive at your muscles as quickly as they need it. You are much less breathless and your muscles will be a good deal less exhausted. This is termed 'aerobic' exercise.

Clearly the type of exercise we recommend to most of our readers (and all of those aged fifty or more) is aerobic. This kind of exercise has been the subject of numerous scientific studies.

Remember the story about the Ancient Briton and the modern office worker? There is a lot of evidence now that exercise and blood fats are closely related. Exercise raises the beneficial HDL-cholesterol and lowers the risky blood triglyceride, while at the same time it burns off calories and helps keep down your weight. There is also evidence that exercise reduces your risk of a heart attack.

For example, an American called Paffenberger showed that Harvard graduates who exercised regularly after leaving college had halved their risk of a heart attack compared to graduates who did not exercise regularly. Here in the UK, Morris performed a famous experiment on bus drivers and bus conductors to show that the drivers, who had sedentary jobs, had a higher risk of heart attack than the conductors, who exercised as part of their job.

We do not recommend that you rush into an exercise programme, but suggest you take it gently and gradually. What will be fine for a relatively fit young woman will not suit an obese sixty-year-old man. But we do believe that anybody, even the disabled – perhaps especially the disabled – will be able to find some kind of regular exercise that will suit them. The best kind of exercises for our purpose use the big muscles of the legs and create a reasonable increase in heart rate. They include light running, jogging and brisk walking. If this kind of exercise causes you pain, for instance angina, we would not recommend it. If all of these are impossible because you are either disabled or have bad angina or your legs are affected by arthritis or intermittent claudication (the cramp caused by narrowing of the arteries to the legs), then light exercise in your local gymnasium or – a really excellent alternative – regular swimming will do the trick.

Remember to start slowly and build up. If running, for instance, only run half a mile or so, run at your ease and stop as often as you need for a breather or to relieve cramps in your legs. A similar build-up principle applies to swimming or gymnasium exercises. It is far more important to discover a kind of exercise you enjoy than to try to force the pace and put yourself in the wrong frame of mind ever after.

Even light regular exercise is beneficial and raises the

HDL-cholesterol – and this has been proved even *after* a heart attack. And there is no age limit to the beneficial effects of regular exercise on blood fats. One suspects that many of the bad effects of ageing are really the bad effects of lifestyle more than the simple consequence of age itself. Fitness is a philosophy for any age. On the other hand smoking almost completely abolishes any benefit you obtain from exercise, a perfect example of how the regime recommended with the Eskimo Diet involves several inter-linked measures rather than reliance on any single measure.

If you have any worry about your fitness to undertake light exercise, have a word with your doctor. Usually this will result in reassurance, and possibly some very useful advice. In a borderline case your doctor may think a medical examination is necessary, with blood tests and an electrocardiogram. If so, take the advice. A knowledge of your own state of health is your right, and it is essential to any planned programme of fitness or exercise.

Alcohol

As we said earlier, we do not condemn alcohol in moderation. Only in large quantities does it act as a poison, especially to the liver, brain and pancreas, but also to the heart. It not only raises the blood fats but directly damages the cells in the heart itself. Although some studies have suggested that alcohol does raise the HDL-cholesterol, it also tends to raise the triglycerides. Taken in excess, it shortens and coarsens the lives of millions; alcohol's calorie content also needs to be considered.

Men should not drink more than two or three pints of beer three times a week. Women should not drink more than two pints or the equivalent three times a week.

Alcohol equivalents

It may surprise many people to discover that a single whisky contains about the same amount of alcohol as half a pint of beer, a small sherry or a glass of wine.

Stress: the hidden menace

What do we mean by stress? For working women and men it will often be competitive pressure in the workplace. For housewives it will revolve about the myriad pressures at home. Some people have the type of personality that naturally leads them into stressful situations; this can as easily be seen in the successful businessman or businesswoman as in the more timid and anxious person whose personality does not lead to great material success.

We have long been aware that if we ask a man or woman at our outpatient clinic if he or she is under stress, the answer these days is almost invariably Yes. It seems we are all under some degree of stress a large part of the time, so it may well be part of normal living. When does it become a threat?

We know when we are under stress because we feel out of sorts. Some people suffer anxiety or bad nerves with symptoms such as a dry mouth, jittery legs, and difficulty with sleeping or concentration. While this may be common at certain times, for instance just before a driving test, if it goes on for long periods there is no question that stress has gone way beyond what might be accepted as normal. Other giveaway symptoms are tension headaches and flying off the emotional handle at little upsets. Perhaps even more common are bowel gripes, abdominal bloating, and aching and tired muscles most of the time, building up especially during the working day. A simple rule of thumb to determine if you are under excess stress is to ask your spouse or a very close relative or friend; they can often see the signs more clearly than you can.

While most of us know when we have been under excessive stress for a long time, it is often surprising how little insight we have into the causes of that stress. Generally speaking, in 90 per cent of working men and women it revolves around the workplace, while for those who do not have a job it revolves around the home.

Does stress lead to heart attacks?

This is the story of one of Dr Ryan's patients whom we shall call John. Suddenly one evening John received a telephone call warning that there was a bomb placed in his grocer's shop. Within only a minute or two he experienced a dull, heavy pain across his chest, making him feel faint and causing him to break into a heavy, cold sweat. He was admitted to hospital within half an hour where the diagnosis was confirmed as a heart attack. This story illustrates how severe acute stress can lead directly to a heart attack. But this type of stress can hardly be predicted and is often unavoidable. In most cases the type of stress that leads to a heart attack is more insidious.

Studies have shown that prolonged stress affects blood fats, raising the total level of blood cholesterol. Of great relevance to the stressed business person and housewife is a study reported to the *American Heart Journal* in 1984 by Meyer Friendman and his colleagues. They investigated an amazing 862 people who had already had one heart attack and were therefore at increased risk of suffering another. These people were divided into two groups: 270 received the standard advice that people are given after a heart attack, while 592 were given counselling on what is called 'type A' behaviour. The researchers followed these people up for a period of three years and observed how frequently they had another heart attack.

A 'type A' personality is a very competitive one characterized by an acute urgency about time so that he or she worries about wasting minutes; this attitude is combined with easily provoked hostility to anybody or anything that gets in the way of his or her perceived notions of efficiency. Sadly, many of us recognize this in ourselves. The staggering finding of this study was that people who were given advice on how to reduce their tendency to 'type A' behaviour had a much lower cumulative risk of a second heart attack (7.2 per cent) compared to the first group, who had not been given this advice (13 per cent).

While other studies have not all proved as clear as this one, there is a general tendency to link stress and increased risk of heart attack. Prolonged stress is bad for us in other ways too – for instance it sometimes plays a part in high blood pressure. But what can we do about it?

Avoiding stress

We have used the term 'avoiding' for good reason. In the majority of cases of prolonged stress, simple common sense will suggest a solution. If the stress is associated with work or the home, you can hardly avoid it, but what you *can* do a great deal about is your reaction to it. We suggest that you sit back for a minute or two and analyse the situations that get you most 'wound up'. It is an excellent idea to get help from your spouse or closest friend. List those situations on a sheet of paper.

Now ask yourself if you can possibly avoid these

situations. If Yes is the answer, do your best to avoid them. If, as we suspect will often be the case, No is the answer, look at the problem with an entirely different perspective.

Say to yourself: usually this winds me up but I am not going to allow it to do so. Take a deep breath, place the cause clearly in your mental sights, then take a mental step backwards from it and reduce its importance to you. These things can usually be put into a completely different perspective – in other words seen not as a vital problem that should have been solved five minutes ago but as a trivial matter that is not going to be allowed to shorten your life. Think of the reaction of your colleagues at work or even more, perhaps, of your family when in the face of such pressure you simply smile.

Other practical techniques to help include the deliberate creation of time during the day to relax, for instance with a cup of tea or light exercise. For many people the opportunity for light exercise will take them completely away from the persistent nagging stress and it will also help reduce their weight and keep their blood fats down.

There will almost certainly be local classes or groups that you can attend. Yoga and meditation may help some, while simpler, Western-based group activities may suit others better. A number of explanatory books and booklets are available to people who need further help in coping with anxiety or stress. These often work best in association with audio tapes, which have the added advantage that you can choose a male or female voice to suit you. Here are just a few:

Dr Robert Sharpe, *Relax and Enjoy It*. This is a very good tape which most people find useful. Available from Lifestyle Training Centre, 23 Abingdon Road, London W3.

For those who prefer a woman's voice: Mary C. Barfield, *Relaxation for Everyday Living*. From 2 Foot Rock

Coastguards, Pett Level, East Sussex, TN35 4EW.

For those who need to practise relaxation alone: *Relaxation and the Management of Stress and Anxiety*. This tape comes with an excellent booklet and it explains how to relate relaxation to everyday situations. From Psychological Counselling Services, 80 Rosemont Road, Liverpool, L17 6DA.

For those who want to read a book about it: H. Selye, *The Stress of Life*, published by McGraw Hill. Alternatives are *Stress and Relaxation* by Jane Madders and *The High Fibre Cookbook* by Pamela Westland, both published by Martin Dunitz.

Raised blood pressure

One very definite way in which stress may undermine your health is by leading to raised blood pressure. Doctors have long been aware of a link between long-term stress and blood pressure. Raised blood pressure in an adult will usually mean a reading of 160/95 mm Hg or higher. In pregnant women, whose blood pressures are much lower than normal due to the opening up of blood vessels in the body by hormones, lower figures than this are still potentially hazardous. The second of the two figures (called the diastolic blood pressure) is taken as the most significant, while the first figure may be very high and not reducible in elderly people who have a very hardened and inelastic aorta. In these circumstances, doctors look to the second figure only.

Over the years in his outpatient clinics, Dr Ryan has seen many cases of what is known as Gaisbock's syndrome. A stressed businessman develops a blood pressure which is initially up and down, termed labile hypertension. As the stress continues over several more years the blood pressure becomes persistently raised.

This is now permanent hypertension, or raised blood pressure. There are many other ways in which blood pressure may become permanently raised, in particular by a lifetime's excessive intake of table salt in somebody who has a family tendency to blood pressure, and in people with a history of kidney disease. But whatever the cause of the blood pressure, once established it is one of the proven risk factors for increasing your liability to a heart attack.

How do you know if you have high blood pressure? Here the public is completely misinformed. Often people will remark that they know their blood pressure is up because they suffer headaches or their face is flushed. This is complete nonsense. Most people who have undiagnosed high blood pressure have no symptoms at all.

In the majority of people with mild to moderate hypertension, the headaches and dizziness tend to come on when people *know* they have high blood pressure. In these people high blood pressure can only be spotted as part of a routine medical examination. That isn't to say that very severe high blood pressure will not provoke symptoms. Fortunately this highly dangerous type of hypertension is relatively rare. Doctors talk about hypertension as the great deceiver, because if you wait for real symptoms it is rather a case of closing the stable door after the horse has bolted. Hypertension puts you at increased risk of a heart attack or a stroke, and is best dealt with by having regular routine medical examinations.

The approach to raised blood pressure is a very simple one. First you try to prevent it (especially if there is a positive history of it in your family or if you have had temporary raised blood pressure during pregnancy – called pre-eclampsia or toxaemia of pregnancy) by reducing long-term stress on yourself and by keeping your salt intake reasonably low. This does not, however, mean no salt at all (see Chapter 8). Routine medical check-ups will diagnose raised blood pressure very early, at which stage it is quite easy to treat with appropriate advice and medication from your family doctor. If you know you have raised blood pressure, don't try any fringe medical treatments. It is a simple condition to manage in most people, yet its long-term consequences if not controlled can be serious. If you do suffer from raised blood pressure, and it is treated in time, it should be possible to reduce it entirely to normal and remove that risk.

Coffee and tea

There is a lot of evidence that the caffeine content of these beverages can induce a state of hyperstimulation, similar to the jitteriness that goes with anxiety. Properly conducted scientific studies have shown that intake of caffeine in coffee particularly may be associated with an increased risk of coronary heart disease. But all this evidence is from relatively few studies and we are not entirely convinced at present that caffeine is a proven risk factor. A high intake can cause other problems, however, so it is as well to cut down.

Once again we would advise a balanced common-sense approach. If you like tea and coffee, there is no medical reason why you shouldn't continue to enjoy it. But it would be wise to cut down to about four cups (of both combined) a day. For many people this will be quite enough. However, if you drink far in excess of this, you should find another drink that you can sometimes take instead of tea or coffee. Often all we need is a hot, appetizing drink rather than the stimulant effect of the caffeine content, so decaffeinated coffee or tea will do. A pleasant alternative is fruit squash with boiling water.

One orange squash will taste quite different from another because of the addition of sweeteners. Experiment with several brands until you find one that suits you.

Sugar – pure white menace or pure white innocence?

In recent years sugar has tended to be seen as a danger to health. The subject remains controversial today, when some authorities see the main problems arising from sugar as obesity and bad teeth. This can lead to other problems which increase the risk of heart attack and diabetes. Our simple advice is that sugar in itself is not a forbidden food but that, to avoid becoming overweight and possibly suffering any further complications, keep it under reasonable control.

Oral contraceptives (the Pill)

We are all aware that the Pill has been linked to a slightly increased tendency to clots within the blood vessels and even to an increase in the risk of heart attack or stroke. The precise degree of risk remains somewhat controversial, but the large number of women taking it safely, together with the modern lower doses of hormones in oral contraceptives, clearly signify that it is only a slight risk. The risk is made worse if you smoke or if you have high blood pressure.

Authors' Afterword

'If thou examinest a man for illness in his cardia [chest], and he has pains in his arm, in his breast and in one side of his cardia... then thou shalt say thereof: it is due to something entering into the mouth, it is death that threatens him.' This is the most extraordinary reference we have ever read to heart attack. It is quoted from the Egyptian medical text called the Papyrus Ebers, and was written 1550 years BC. We are indebted to our colleague, consultant surgeon Mr John Rowling, for drawing our attention to it.

Nothing could better encapsulate the description of the pain of heart attack or the vital importance of diet in its cause. It has taken us three thousand five hundred years to come back to that same understanding as a priest-doctor on the banks of the Nile!

While some will undoubtedly find that this confirms their superstition that heart attacks are a 'natural' phenomenon, and that you can therefore do nothing about them, we would point out equally cogently that tuberculosis too was a common disease in Ancient Egypt and there is nothing natural about it – it is caused by a deadly bacterium. Heart attacks are the result of disease and not natural processes. So what is the good news?

Modern science has given us the means to fight back hard against this fearsome killer. And our first weapon against it is understanding.

We can begin this process of saving ourselves by appreciating just what a heart attack is. A heart attack results from a long accumulation of insults within the arteries to our hearts. It has taken western science an astonishingly long time to confirm the belief of the Ancient Egyptians: the avenues of entry for these insults are our mouths. We don't guarantee that if you take the advice given in this book you won't have a heart attack. But by understanding the processes, from the earliest fatty streaks of the arteries of children through to the final clot in hardened and grossly diseased atheromatous coronary arteries of our middle and old age, we can take active and relatively simple measures which will cut the risk of our dying of a heart attack to a minimum.

Our aim in writing this book was to reveal to the general public the new knowledge in the field of heart attack prevention. We hope we will have achieved some good from writing it. In Britain the public has lagged behind its counterparts in much of the western world in its awareness of many of the facts we have given you here. The result has been a lesser decline in the number of people suffering heart attacks in the UK when compared to other western countries such as the United States, Canada, Australia and Scandinavia.

If there is a single simple message we would like to close with, it is this: Don't regard a heart attack as bad luck or an act of fate. It's a disease like any other disease – and you can do a great deal to prevent it. Don't wait for it to happen. Use knowledge and understanding to do something positive about preventing it. There is no other way to win – and we can and will win this medical battle.

Good health!

Dr Reg Saynor and Dr Frank Ryan

Useful Addresses

The British Heart Foundation is an organization that is specifically interested in advising patients on how to cope with a heart attack. They also advise people on how best to cope with heart surgery, blood pressure and raised blood fats, and they support a good deal of the cardiac research that is performed throughout the United Kingdom. This charitable organization has branches throughout the UK and will provide advice and free literature to anybody who contacts them.

If you wish to know more about them or would like their advice, or if you wish to help with research into heart disease, send a stamped self-addressed envelope to:

British Heart Foundation
102 Gloucester Place
London W1H 4DH

Action on Smoking and Health (ASH)
5–11 Mortimer Street
London W1N 7RH

National Society of Non–Smokers (QUIT)
Latimer House
40–48 Hanson Street
London W1P 7DE

Health Education Authority
Hamilton House
Mabledon Place
London WC1H 9TX

For advice on resuscitation classes go to your local Health Education Unit. Failing this try:

Margaret Willis
Sheffield Health Education Unit
119 Manchester Road
Sheffield S10

Also for training in resuscitation:

St John's Ambulance
Head Office
1 Grosvenor Cresent
London SW1X 7EF

For advice on fish-oil products:

Seven Seas Health Care Ltd
Marfleet
Kingston-upon-Hull
HU9 5NJ

Remember, if you wish to receive advice booklets, to send a large stamped addressed envelope.

List of Useful Terms

Adrenalin — hormone-producing adrenal gland which is secreted at time of stress, danger or serious illness.

Angina — see p. 21

Angioplasty — see p. 46

Anticoagulant — see p. 73

Arrhythmia — disordered beat or heart rhythm.

Artery — thick-walled blood vessel which carries oxygenated blood from the heart to the tissues of the body, with the exception of the pulmonary artery which carries deoxygenated blood from the heart to the lungs.

Atheroma — see p. 20

Atheromatous plaques — see p. 21

Blood pressure — the pressure of blood in the arteries, expressed as two figures. The upper figure is called the systolic, the lower figure diastolic. See page 177.

CABG or cabbage grafting — see p. 44

Calorie — unit of energy. Usually expressed as kilocalories (kcal) when applied to energy intake from food. Alternative expression is kilojoules, (kJ). 1 kcal = 4.184 (kJ). Different foods give different energy yields, ie, 1 g carbohydrate = 3.75 kcal, 1 g fat = 9 kcal, 1 g protein = 4 kcal, 1 g alcohol = 7 kcal.

Carbohydrate — food derived from sugar. If one molecule of carbohydrate is made up from one molecule of sugar, it is a monosaccharide, like sucrose; many molecules of sugar it is a polysaccharide, like starch.

Cholesterol — see p. 53

Claudication — cramp-like pain in the leg muscle on walking, caused by narrowing of the arteries to the legs.

Electrocardiogram (ecg) — a record on paper of the heart's electrical cycle. Used in diagnosis of angina, heart attack, or arrhythmia.

Fatty acids — see p. 60
Fibrinogen — see pp. 25 and 73
HDL-cholesterol — see p. 49
Hydrogenated/hydrolized fats — see p. 61
Ischaemic — suffering for want of blood, as in ischaemic heart disease, heart disease due to narrowed coronary arteries.
LDL-cholesterol — see p. 49
Monounsaturated fats — see p. 61
Pacemaker — the heart has its own natural pacemaker called the sino-atrial node. This can be replaced by an artificial pacemaker in people where the sino-atrial node is faulty.
Peptic Ulcer — Acid-related ulcer in the duodenum, stomach or gullet.
Platelets — see pp. 25 and 30
Polyunsaturated fats — see p. 61
Protein — complicated molecule vital to body function made up from chemicals called amino acids.
Red blood cells — discs containing haemoglobin, which transport oxygen in the blood. As they are full of oxygen, the blood is oxygenated (in the arteries); if oxygen is used up, they are deoxygenated (in the vein).
Saturated fats — see p. 61
Stroke — sudden damage to the brain as a result of either a blocked artery or a bleed into the substance of the brain (cerebral haemorrhage).
Tachycardia — see p. 169
Thrombolytic therapy — see p. 42
Triglyceride — see p. 57
Vascular disease — disease of an internal organ caused by either a narrowing or blocking of the artery to it or rupture of a blood vessel within it, ie heart attack, angina, stroke, intermittent claudication.
Vein — thin-walled blood vessel, carrying deoxygenated blood back to the heart (except the pulmonary veins, which carry oxygenated blood back from the lungs to the heart).
Ventricular fibrillation — life-threatening disorder of the electrical control of the heartbeat. In effect the heart is stopped.
White blood cells — living cells in the blood which fight infection and play a vital part in inflammation.

Index